The Fungus Link

An Introduction to
Fungal Disease

Including the Initial Phase Diet

by

Doug A. Kaufmann

Compilation Edited by

Beverly Thornhill Hunt, Ph.D.

MediaTrition
Rockwall, Texas

Published by MediaTrition
301 W. Washington Street
Rockwall, Texas 75087
972-772-0990

Publisher's Cataloging-in-Publication
(provided by Quality Books, Inc.)

Kaufmann, Doug A., 1949-
   The fungus link : an introduction to fungal disease,
including the initial phase diet / by Doug A. Kaufmann ;
edited by Beverly Thornhill Hunt. – 1st ed.
   p. cm.
   Includes bibliographical references and index.
   ISBN: 0-9703418-0-6

   1. Mycoses – Popular works. 2. Medical mycology –
Popular works. 3. Pathogenic fungi.   I. Title

RC117.K38 2000   616.9'69'071
                                        QB100-784

This book is dedicated to...

...the living and deceased patients
erroneously diagnosed with a serious
disease when all the while they were
actually suffering from an undiagnosed
fungal condition, and

...the open-minded physicians who help
the sick and prevent pain, suffering, and
death by treating every symptom and
disease of unknown etiology as though it
was due to fungus.
Your peers will scoff, but
your patients will flourish.

Foreword

I have known Doug Kaufmann for many years, have had many patients in common with him, and have come to respect his work as a nutritionist and as a fungal expert. In this book, you will read practical information about what fungal illness is, how common a health problem it is, how to recognize it by its symptoms, and how to eradicate it from the body. The testimonials presented give strong support to the seriousness and frequency of fungal illness as a human health problem. I, too, have seen in my own practice fungi representing the primary underlying cause of diverse health conditions including chronic fatigue syndrome, crippling arthritis, severe intestinal disorders, chronic allergies, chronic respiratory illness, "brain fog" syndrome, depression, and chronic skin conditions (eczema, psoriasis, pruritic dermatitis). The sections written by other health professionals prove that fungal illness is being recognized by more and more doctors for its serious impact on human health.

If you or someone you love has a chronic illness, read this book thoroughly. Next, reflect on or pray about what you have read. Then strongly consider changing your diet (or the diet of your loved one) for a few weeks to starve the fungi (as described in the appendix). Even consider taking some anti-fungal herbals (also described in the appendix) or prescription anti-fungal medications if you can find a doctor who will assist you. When you do these things and you initially feel worse (described in this book as the Herxheimer "die off" reaction) then days later feel better than you have in a long time, you probably had fungi causing much of your illness. Become proactive, take charge of your own health, and seek out a health practitioner who understands the effect of fungal illness and related conditions on your health. Read, learn, implement what you learn, and be well!

Wm. Lee Cowden, M. D.

co-author: *Alternative Medicine*
Definitive Guide to Cancer and
Cancer Diagnosis: What To Do Next

Preface

In 1996, Dr. David Holland and I were busy gathering data to confirm our suspicions that what we had been observing clinically had scientific validity. For the previous 25 years, I had been able to assist people with many diseases and symptoms by addressing a germ that physicians had completely missed in their diagnoses. There are today approximately 80 documented autoimmune diseases, each one without an etiological basis (known cause). Scientists have no idea what causes the heart attacks and cancers that kill one million people annually. In medicine, the word "germ" is often used synonymously with the word "bacteria." This, in a small way, illustrates the confusion regarding the causes of disease among even the brightest medical practitioners and scientists.

So it is that the first book we know of to implicate fungus as the cause of debilitation and death has been completed. As you peruse these pages, know that this work includes scientific notation and confirmation of the hypothesis that disease *does* have a known pathogen and is *not* bacterial in every instance!

I suppose the invention of antibiotics was viewed as revolutionary by those in 1950s science. Our brightest, best scientists concluded that we had finally defeated the germs responsible for causing sickness and disease. If this were true, 1955 should have been a banner year in science. Certainly those millions who took antibiotics in that five year time span were now less vulnerable to common maladies. If not, they reasoned, then perhaps more antibiotics would permanently fix them. I have often used the analogy of calcium intake and osteoporosis in America to prove my point before surrendering to the notion that antibiotics were not the magic bullet hoped for. If osteoporosis were due to calcium deficiency, Americans would never have osteoporosis. Today, celebrity white moustaches abound, beckoning us to drink more milk! Between the calcium supplements we throw down our throats and the amount of milk that we drink, our bones should never become fragile!

Yet the opposite is true in each of these situations. Osteoporosis is striking more Americans than ever before in history, despite dairy intake and calcium supplementation. Bacteria continue to elude even the best antibiotics, despite the billions of dollars of pharmaceutical research. Unless the etiology (cause) of a disease is identified, all the supplements and drugs in the world may be for naught.

Early in the year 2000, researchers discovered that the density of the bones of laboratory mice improved up to 50 percent when they were given cholesterol-lowering drugs. It is even more important to note that cholesterol-lowering drugs are antifungal medications. That brings us full circle.

This book is a compilation of data originally published from 1997 to 1999 in *The Fungazette* -- our early attempt at what, today, is a very successful newsletter. This book and our current newsletter help our readers locate the possible cause of their health maladies. It seems an especially lonely existence when you are sick and no one knows why. This book does not replace the diagnosis, prognosis, or treatment that your health care practitioner can provide. But it is my hope that, in time, the competency at diagnosing fungal disease will improve. I can assure you that will happen if medical protocol will call for proper diet and antifungal herbs or medicines for their difficult patients. There is nothing more convincing than observing life threatening diseases frequently respond favorably to simple antifungal therapy.

BIOGRAPHIES

Doug A. Kaufmann is the founder of Kaufmann Nutrition Center. He daily hosts the popular nationally-syndicated radio program *The Doug Kaufmann Health Show* on USA Radio Network and the television program *Your Health with Doug Kaufmann* on FamilyNet. His extensive medical background began in 1969 while training as a U. S. Navy Corpsman. Doug served in that capacity in Vietnam and has continued his medical education for the past 28 years. His background encompasses laboratory, research, and clinical nutrition. His 1984 book, *The Food Sensitivity Diet*, was in print for eight years and can still be found in libraries.

David A. Holland, M.D. completed his Bachelor of Science with a major in Microbiology at Texas Tech University. In 1993, he graduated from Texas Tech University Health Science Center with his doctorate degree. Dr. Holland completed his internship in General Practice in Fort Worth, Texas. During his residency, he met and began studying fungal diseases with Doug Kaufmann. Dr. Holland learned that nutritional intervention frequently prevented the onset of serious disease and also played a role in its reversal. He is currently completing a residency in family practice.

Patrick Kwan, MSc. received his BSc. in Microbiology at the University of California, Riverside. He also graduated with a MSc. from Oregon State University. Mr. Kwan is a founding member of Diversified Research, the largest food laboratory in Canada. For 13 years, he was a senior consultant to George Weston, Ltd., the largest retail food chain in Canada.

<u>Milt Gearing, Ph.D.</u> received his doctorate from the University of South Carolina in clinical psychology. Dr. Gearing was formerly director of Psychological Services of Charter Hospital of Dallas.

<u>Nathan L. Lipton, M.D.</u> is a Fellow, American Academy of Ophthalmologists, and Diplomate, American Board of Ophthalmology.

<u>C. R. Mabray, M.D.</u> is a Fellow in the American College of Obstetricians and Gynecologists.

<u>Richard Becker, D.O.</u> has been 15 years in family practice. He received his B.A. in biochemistry from Loma Linda University, a world leader in nutritional therapies, and his graduate degree from the Health Science College of Osteopathic Medicine in Kansas City, Missouri. Dr. Becker is a Hodgkins lymphoma survivor and follows Doug Kaufmann's nutritional approach to the treatment of cancer.

Table of Contents

Chapter Four

Relating Fungus to Respiration

Chapter Five

Relating Fungus to Brain Disorders
and Mental Health

APPENDIX A
The Initial Phase Diet
by Doug A. Kaufmann

APPENDIX B
Product Information

INDEX

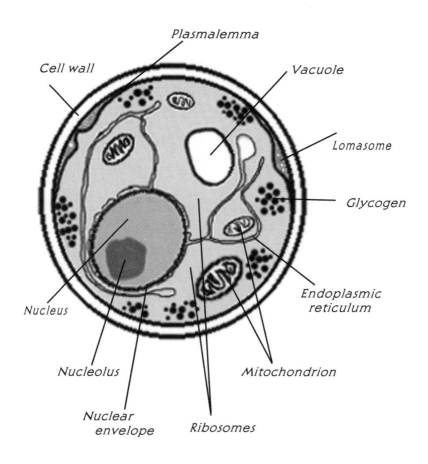

Plasmalemma

Cell wall

Vacuole

Lomasome

Glycogen

Endoplasmic
reticulum

Nucleus

Nucleolus

Mitochondrion

Nuclear
envelope

Ribosomes

Diagram of a cross section of a generalized
fungus cell

FUNGUS

A simple plant that lacks
chlorophyll.
Fungi include the yeasts,
rust, molds, and mushrooms.
They live as either saprophytes
or parasites of plants and
animals (man).
Some species infect
and cause disease
in man.

- The Bantam Medical Dictionary

Chapter One

Relating Fungus to Your Health

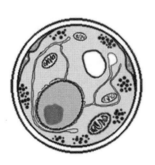

A Doctor's Introduction to Nutrition and Fungus

by Roby Mitchell, Ph.D., M.D.

Greetings to all of you! I want to congratulate you for taking the time to educate yourself on being an active participant in improving your health. You are, potentially, the best doctor you could ever have.

I'd like to begin by introducing myself to you and letting you know how Doug and I became associated. My background is in traditional western medicine. I graduated with honors from Texas Tech School of Medicine. Subsequently, I started a practice as an emergency room physician. The emergency room is the epitome of acute care medicine, so I saw lots of patients suffering from symptoms of diseases that had not been adequately addressed for years. Many fell under the category of vascular disease, which includes "heart attack" and stroke. These problems develop after years of investing in lifestyle choices that clog up the arteries of the heart and brain.

What made me begin to question the way I practiced medicine was the number of young people, 45 to 60, that came in to the emergency room with these problems. It is tragic to go out into the waiting room and tell a family that their loved one is dead, but it is oppressively heartrending when it is a relatively young mother and her children who have just lost their husband, father, and breadwinner.

3

Reading the medical literature of the time also engendered some discomfort, as it was reporting that upwards of 80% of these tragic events were completely preventable by implementing some relatively simple lifestyle changes. I was telling that young mother and her children that "we did all that we could do," but obviously that was not the case.

During my medical school training, I was chosen to participate in a student exchange program between Texas Tech and Jinan University in Canton, China. There I studied Chinese traditional medicine, which included the use of foods, herbal medicines, and acupuncture to treat disease. Their philosophy focused on getting the whole body system back into balance and allowing the body's intelligence to do the healing. The physician was an assistant or facilitator. I was starting to wonder if this was not a more appropriate way to reestablish health.

Coincidental with these ruminations was the release of a study done by Dr. Dean Ornish. He had proven that you could open up clogged arteries by implementing a regime of exercise, stress reduction, and healthful eating. This could save millions in health care costs each year and prevent patients from undergoing the risks and trauma of surgical procedures.

Seeing more and more MDs start to adopt this philosophy, I started a little sideline practice that focused on teaching patients lifestyle changes instead of always relying on medications. Once the word got out that there was an M.D. in Amarillo, Texas, who focused on natural healing, my phone started ringing off the wall. I found myself spending more time in this type of practice, even though I also continued my E.R. practice. This led to my doing a self-study course on nutrition and its link to disease. I learned how nutrients from plant sources were being used to prevent and treat many diseases.

During my investigations, I ran across a product called Juice Plus that was being touted as being the alternative to juicing. I had never taken supplements in the past, but I knew that I was not getting the recommended amount of raw fruits and vegetables in my diet. I was so impressed after having this product analyzed that I started taking it. Within two to three weeks, I felt increased energy, improved quality of sleep, improved regularity, and my recovery time after workouts decreased (I participate in triathlons). I had similarly impressive results with my mom, dad, and other family members. It wasn't long before I, who had been staunchly anti-vitamin mineral supplementation, was being asked to speak across the United States, Canada, and Europe on the benefits of these whole food capsules that replaced juicing several pounds of organic fruits and organic vegetables.

One of the places I was asked to speak was on a then little-known health talk show hosted by who else? Doug Kaufmann. Doug and I became fast friends as we shared similar convictions about the role of individual responsibility in health care and the benefits of nutritional supplements in preventing and treating diseases. I also found Doug to share a similar skepticism and integrity. He had also investigated Juice Plus and recommended it to some of his clients.

Fortunately for me, Doug became not only a friend but also a mentor. I'm relatively new at practicing the type of medicine that Doug has been espousing and training other medical professionals in for over 20 years. So far, the most important lesson he has taught me is the association of a wide variety of clinical syndromes with systemic (all over the body) candidiasis, commonly known as yeast.

This has been a much-maligned diagnosis in the past because it has eluded laboratory verification. However, because of the scientific verification Doug presented to me, as well as the trust I had developed in his clinical expertise, I started treating patients who fit the yeast profile. A combination of prescriptive antifungals, a diet devoid of refined sugars and yeasts, immune system enhancement with Juice Plus, and replacement of "good" intestinal bacteria genuinely helped these patients.

The results have been nothing short of miraculous for many patients. Many had suffered for years with symptoms of chronic fatigue, PMS, depression, irritable bowel, obesity, attention deficit disorder, asthma, interstitial cystitis, bladder incontinence, prostatitis, psoriasis, MS, and fibromyalgia. They dramatically improved if they followed the treatment protocol.

I can't thank Doug enough for teaching me about this life-changing therapy. My patients would thank him, too, if they knew that he was responsible for teaching me. However, in order to maintain my status as a near-deity, I am forced to keep that a secret!

6

What the Experts Say about Fungal Diseases

by Doug A. Kaufmann

There is certainly no shortage of scientific literature about fungal symptoms and diseases. And the twentieth century holds nothing as far as knowledge of the many diseases caused by fungus. Just open a Bible and go directly to Leviticus 14 verses 34 and 35. This talk of fungus causing health problems is not new.

As far as twentieth century fungal experts, consider Dr. Lida Mattman, a professor emeritus at Wayne State university. In her excellent book *Stealth Pathogens,* Dr. Mattman asks, "Are fungi in blood smears overlooked because they are confused with blood cells?" She answers a resounding, "Yes!" From that one statement alone, just imagine how many blood conditions are misdiagnosed because machines or laboratory technologists just can't differentiate between spores and cells.

Another bold statement is made on the same page. This one by Dr. M. G. Rinaldi, who says, "Given the right immunocompromised host, virtually any fungus can kill a human being."

David Holland, M.D., has a book in his office called *Medical Mycology* by C. C. Kibbler. (Mycology is the study of fungus.) In this book, published in 1995, 18 prominent physicians from large research universities like Duke, Texas University, and

Stanford expound on the serious health threats that fungi pose. Here are some of the chapters in *Medical Mycology*: Fungal Disease of the Bone and Joint; Fungal Diseases of the Cardio-vascular System; Mycoses [fungi] causing mass lesions of the Central Nervous System; Fungal Diseases in Dermatology; Fungal Infections of the Ear, Nose, and Throat; Fungal Infections of the Gastrointestinal Tract; Fungal Infections of the Respiratory Tract; and even Fungal Diseases in Opthalmology. Wouldn't you think every doctor in the world would understand that these microorganisms might cause disease? Why don't they? I am glad you asked!

Most doctors believe that fungus only infects immunocompromised (lowered immunity) patients. If this were true, then San Joaquin Valley Fever, caused by breathing the fungi Coccidioides immitus, could not have possibly killed young, healthy military men. What about the ABC episode of *Primetime* aired April 9, 1997, dealing with infants who are sick and dying from fungal exposure in their homes? Or are women who suffer from vaginal yeast infections immuno-compromised? In each of these instances, the integrity of the immune system was only challenged AFTER fungal exposure – not before. So, who is immunocompromised? Are the air we breathe and the water we drink compromising our immune systems? How about the medicines that most Americans take? Since antibiotics are mycotoxins (fungal poisons), perhaps we can now define compromised immunity as applying to anyone who has ever taken an antibiotic! That is certainly a lot of people, but while you ponder that potential statistic, the following may put it in perspective for you.

In 1963, Dr. Harold T. Hyman published in *The Complete Home Medical Encyclopedia* that approximately one-half of the population of the United States had, at one time or another, suffered from a fungal disorder that had been "unrecognized." Now, my question for you is: has medical science really progressed since 1963? Or are 125,000,000 Americans still suffering from "unrecognized" fungal disorders?

Asking Doug and Dave

by Doug Kaufmann and Dr. David A. Holland

Q On your radio shows, I hear you talk about fungus as the cause of many health problems. If this is true, why don't doctors know about this? WM, Vancouver, WA

A You can imagine how many times we hear this question every day! We feel that the primary reason doctors don't understand the role of fungus in the disease process is lack of education. Not that your doctor is not educated, just the opposite is true. Fungal infections were very rare 50 years ago. In medicine, tradition is extremely valuable and breaking tradition does not often occur. Such is the case with fungal diseases.

Frankly, the reason that fungal infections were rare 50 years ago is because the pharmaceutical drugs that cause fungal infections were also rare or non-existent. To illustrate this point, in the April, 1996, issue of *Healthweek* magazine, writer Mary Ann Hellinghausen addressed the very question you have. The headline read: **Fungal Infections Pose Dangers**. In this article, Dr. Michael G. Rinaldi stated, "We can't neglect fungal diseases any longer." Dr. Rinaldi went on to explain what we already know in our clinic: we just didn't see fungus infections 50 years ago. Why? Because we didn't have drugs that contributed to fungal growth! According to Dr. Rinaldi, "We're using antibiotics that are so powerful they save lives, but they also destroy normal flora, particularly in our intestinal tract. This allows pathogenic germs to colonize and eventually become infectious." Such is the case with fungal pathogens! It may take another decade, but more and more doctors are now recognizing not only the benefits but also the dangers inherent in prescriptive drugs.

Q I have asthma and have heard that even this can be caused by fungus. How do I tell if this is the case? JM, Dallas, TX

A Do you remember when your asthma started? Was it following antibiotic, cortisone, or birth control pill usage? Although not exclusively due to these drugs, *bronchio pulmonary fungi* are sometimes misdiagnosed as asthma. A condition called farmers lung may also appear to be asthma. With symptoms that are similar, even the brightest of asthma specialists miss fungus as the real root of some of these cases. Systemic antifungal drugs that would get into the lungs and eradicate fungus can be tried. Ask your doctor about these.

Q Can fungi affect the brain? CM, Bangor, ME

A Yes, fungus can impregnate brain tissue, and such conditions are grave in that fungus can proliferate quickly and cause death. Since the inception of antibiotics, numerous publications have spoken about a condition called "meningeal fungi."

In Chapter 5 we expound on this phenomenon of fungi within the tissues surrounding the brain possibly causing aberrant behavior. Dr. A. V. Costantini is publishing that hyperactivity may have its roots in mycotoxins (fungal poisons). If this is the case, it is highly likely that other brain malfunctions may also be due to fungi.

Q How does fungus get into our bodies? Do we eat fungus? BB, Portland, OR

A Let's answer your second question first. In a book called *Industrial Microbiology* there is a list of foods that ferment. The fermentation of foods takes place in the presence of fungi. For example, the fungus Rhizopus ferments soybeans into tempeh. Soybean is a relatively common food in the American diet. Then one must consider the food chain when concerning ourselves with fungi in our diet. The fungal poison aflatoxin B1 is one of the most deadly poisons known to exist. Corn, stored in warm, moist, mildewing silos, can become impregnated with this deadly fungus. Government regulations prohibit human consumption of corn infested with aflatoxin B1, but they don't prohibit animals from consuming it! Corn infested with 300 parts per billion is fed to chickens and cattle. And who eats the chickens and cattle? You get the picture!

Another way fungus enters our systems is through contact with the soil. For those of you who like to garden, a cut or abrasion on the skin opens a passageway for soil-based fungi. Let's not forget that once fungi have gained access to our bodies, drugs like antibiotics, cortisone, and birth control pills can either initiate or exacerbate fungal proliferation. This is sometimes dangerous given that their fuel is the standard American diet (SAD!).

Chapter Two

Relating Fungus to Arthritis

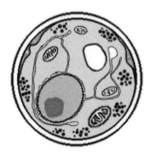

Arthritis: The Fungus Connection

by David Holland, M.D.

The painful fact (no pun intended) about most forms of arthritis is that, with the exception of some infectious arthritis conditions, the cause is unknown. For example, the Arthritis Foundation describes rheumatoid arthritis as a "chronic, systemic, inflammatory disorder of unknown etiology."[1] Etiology simply means "the cause or origin" of a disease.

What does fungus have to do with arthritis? First, we'll read what several doctors have to say about the connection, and then we will visit, first hand, the story of one of our patients. Fungi can cause arthritis by either infecting a joint directly, usually spreading via the blood from the primary infection (e.g., the lungs or intestines), or they may indirectly affect a joint by giving off fungal poisons or "mycotoxins." When this happens, several different types of arthritis may occur.

Let's start with gout. Nearly every medical school in the country teaches that gout is caused by uric acid which, when reaching critical levels, forms crystals in the joints. These crystals cause inflammation and are followed by excruciating pain. Dr. A. V. Costantini, M.D., retired head of the World Health Organization (WHO) Center for Mycotoxins in Food, disagrees. At a 1994 symposium held in Toronto, Canada, Dr. Costantini presented a series of studies by fellow researchers showing that we can't prove that the human body can even manufacture uric acid. In fact, he said, uric acid in the blood stream is more likely of fungal origin.[2] It is the result of fungus entering the body from outside. Furthermore, the studies showed that the urate crystals found in patients with gout occurred days after the inflammation had already set in! Urate crystals were not the cause of the pain experienced by gout patients. So sure was Dr. Costantini of this research that he offered $1,000 to anyone who could prove that the human body created uric acid. As of today, he is not a penny poorer!

Now, let's examine rheumatoid arthritis. In the January 1995 edition of *The Townsend Letter for Doctors*, 19 doctors wrote that a condition known as candidiasis (from the yeast Candida albicans) could mimic symptoms associated with rheumatoid arthritis.[3] Dr. O. Truss, M.D., one of the authors, explained that fungus may play the leading role in symptoms and diseases such as allergies, gastrointestinal and bladder problems, fatigue, weight gain, and even "brain symptoms" like head-aches, poor concentration, and irritability. Dr. Costantini's work also found evidence that mycotoxins caused rheumatoid arthritis.[2]

If you have not had success with your arthritis treatment, talk with your physician about this research and request that he or she prescribe any one of the several systemic antifungal medi-cines for a few weeks. While taking these, you must also avoid foods that would feed the fungi in the joints. Simply stop eating sugars (including those in dairy products, oranges, and melons), potatoes, and beans (including peanuts) for a month or two. If successful, you might want to terminate the drugs and try herbal antifungal remedies. Either way, your success will demonstrate to you and your doctor that the cause of *your* arthritis is no longer listed as "unknown."

References
1. Schumacher, H. Ralph, Jr., M.D. (Ed.). *Primer on the Rheumatic Diseases* (9th Ed.). The Arthritis Foundation. Atlanta, Georgia. 1988.
2. Costantini, A. V., M.D. *The Fungal Mycotoxin Etiology of Human Disease*. Johann Friedrich Oberlin Verlag. Freiburg, Germany. and
   Costantini, A. V., M.D., *The Fungal Mycotoxin Conference*. Toronto, Canada. 1994
3. Brown, Raymond Keith, M.D., et. al. Candidiasis: The Scourge of Arthritics. *The Townsend Letter for Doctors*. 911 Tyler Street, Port Townsend, Washington, 98368-6541. January 1995.

"Healthy Days are Here Again!"

A Testimonial
by Debbie O., Dallas, Texas

Our daughter, Julie, was diagnosed with bacterial meningitis when she was 14 months old. It is common with this kind of meningitis for infection to settle in the joints. In Julie's case, it was her left elbow that was to be infected. After 14 days at the hospital on intravenous antibiotics, we finally came home ready to forget the previous three weeks. Fortunately, Julie returned to our family as a happy, healthy little girl, with the exception of a total hearing loss in one ear. Each year we saw an orthopedic doctor to be certain that the infection, and her slightly enlarged elbow, did not abnormally affect the growth of her arm.

All was well for ten years. After turning 11, Julie began to complain that her elbow was sore. We assumed that this pain was related to a change in the weather, or a bump, or a fall. Several days passed with no improvement, and we decided to make an appointment with an orthopedic doctor. After observation, X-rays, and Advil for a few weeks, it was decided that she should have an MRI.

The results of the MRI determined that Julie suffered from synovitis, which is a condition where fluid collects in the sac surrounding the elbow joint. The recovery and rehabilitation were very slow, painful, and frustrating for an 11-year-old and her parents. Unfortunately, the doctors were never able to determine what caused the inflammation in the elbow.

Just when we thought rehabilitating the elbow would mark an end to our ordeal, Julie began experiencing joint stiffness in different areas of her body. Most of the pain was in her neck, right index finger, and right ankle; however, some days her knee or her hip would also bother her. The stiffness, besides limiting her physical activity, affected her emotionally. Needless to say, we were worried and frightened by this unexplainable condition.

After another trip to the doctor, countless questions, blood tests, and a visit to a pediatric rheumatologist, she was diagnosed with juvenile rheumatoid arthritis. We followed conventional medical advice and through many tears, conversations, and lots of reading, decided to put Julie on a non-steroidial anti-inflammatory drug. Unfortuantely, it did not help. It was then suggested that we "needed to be more aggressive with our approach." The next step was a more potent anti-inflammatory and gold injections. Everything we read made us more disheartened and disappointed. What we were reading and hearing made us think that we would be doing more harm than good.

It was at that point that we made a desperation call to Doug Kaufmann at Nutrition Resources. A friend of ours had mentioned Doug's work and encouraged us to call him. After talking with Doug on the phone for a few minutes, he gave us our first real hope since our personal nightmare began.

After visiting with Julie, Doug and Dr. David Holland told us that her problems might be yeast related. Dr. Holland prescribed an antifungal medicine and placed Julie on a restrictive diet. After two weeks, she felt 99% better. Once again, Julie was able to walk around easily and resume her normal physical activities, pain free. Most importantly to us, she donned her sweet smile. Julie continued on the diet for another month and, while it was not easy, it sure beat the alternatives! For the first time in seven months, Julie felt and acted like a happy, healthy 11-year-old – thanks to the wise counsel and common sense advice from Doug and Dr. Dave.

Chapter Three

Relating Fungus to Digestion

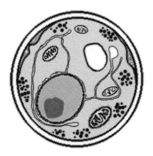

Intestinal Disorders and Fungus

by Doug A. Kaufmann

As the title indicates, I am expounding on intestinal problems in this section. There are those of us who feel that seemingly harmless prescriptive drugs (i.e., antibiotics, cortisone, and birth control pills) can alter the terrain of the bowel enough to initiate an intestinal yeast infection. So often the intestines are the first tissues that are damaged by these activated yeasts, or fungi. For that reason, I thought you should learn how to identify whether your gut problems are really a serious disease for which you are relegated to a life of medicines, or whether your doctor may have been unaware that intestinal fungus can mimic serious intestinal disorders.

What serious gut diseases can these gut yeast infections mimic? Of equal importance is that you understand that the portal of entry of these disease initiators is, in this case, the mouth. Not only is there significant evidence that mycotoxins (fungal poisons) occur in our food supply, but once these devious little mold spores become activated (remember, antibiotics can activate them), everyday foods within our diet may feed them and keep them proliferating throughout the intestines. Of course, once flourishing within our intestines they can make life miserable. In these cases, it is quite common to have bloating, belching, intestinal gas, constipation, diarrhea, indigestion, and esophageal reflux. You can imagine what happens when these fungi escape the intestines via a "leaky gut" – a condition that is actually common once these fungi become active in the intestines.

Crohn's disease and irritable bowel syndrome (IBS) are very serious intestinal disorders. The dictionary states that sections of the alimentary (digestive) tract becomes inflamed, thickened, and ulcerated with these diseases. Crohn's disease is also known as *regional enteritis*, as *regional enterocolitis*, and as *inflammatory granulomatous bowel disease*. I will never understand why one set of symptoms had to be called by four different names, but such is allopathic medicine! You do not suppose that a disease so complex as to have four names might actually be a fungus in the gut and not really a disease at all, do you?

Two testimonial letters in this chapter are very thought provoking. I would not say that either case is cured of bowel disease; however, both found significant relief in addressing an underlying fungal condition. I often wonder what would have happened if I had met these people *before* the gastroenterologists met them. Could I have prevented further deterioration of the bowel? Was surgery really necessary? What role did carbohydrates or antibiotics play in the beginnings of their gut problems? More than their wonderful letters, I have begun to love both of these contributors and I thank them for the courage in apprising others of the fungal link to their diseases. Could fungus be contributing to your stomach and intestinal problems also? You bet it could!

The saddest part of these debilitating gut diseases remains that many gastroenterologists have absolutely no idea that there exists a fungal pathology in many cases of Crohn's and ulcerative colitis. By treating a pathogen (fungus) rather than a disease, it is very likely that many patients with gut diseases will get better faster. And most importantly, if a fungal condition exists after a short course of antifungal medicines, the patient can initiate an antifungal herbal approach. You might want the doctor to prescribe a systemic and gut antifungal medicine for a few weeks just to ascertain whether your gut problems are really a serious gut disease or fungus. If you feel better within two to four weeks, get to a health food store and inquire about natural antifungal remedies.

.

"Mycotoxins" - Fungus Found in Food

by Patrick Kwan, M.Sc.

I have been following Doug Kaufmann's theory of the possible linkage between fungi and certain health disorders with interest for several years because I believe that what he says makes a lot of sense. When Doug asked me to write an article for *The Fungazette*, I was slightly taken aback and jokingly asked him, "What does a food scientist know about fungi?"

Doug replied, "You must have a lot of dealings with molds and yeasts in your work with food products. Just think about it. I'm certain that you know more about fungi than you think."

After pondering Doug's suggestion for a while, I decided that Doug was right. I do deal with mold and fungus in my business … or should I say it deals with me!

I almost got into medical mycology (the study of fungus) when I first started graduate school years ago. I was already a licensed medical technologist specializing in microbiology, and it always intrigued me that nobody seemed to be concerned with or knew much about fungi and their relationship to human beings, except for vaginal yeast infections. Partly because I could not find a good mentor in medical mycology, I ended up studying food science.

Back in the early 1970s, *aflatoxin* was one of the growing
concerns for food scientists. It had first come into prominence
in the early 1960s when several flocks of turkeys suffered from
acute *aflatoxin* poisoning in England. Yes, large doses of this
fungal poison can cause death, even in humans! In this case,
over 100,000 turkeys died of *aflatoxin* poisoning. Later,
scientists would learn that the *aflatoxins* that caused the deaths
were traced to peanut meal in the turkeys feed mix. It turned
out that the peanut meal was stored in an old silo with a
window on one side. As the sun beat down on the feed mix
through the windows, evaporation occurred and the resulting
moisture migrated to the cooler side of the silo, away from the
sun. The increased moisture on the cool side then allowed the
mold *Aspergillus flavus* to proliferate and produce the mold
poison called *aflatoxin*. Since that time, much research has
been done on *aflatoxin* and its tumor-causing effects on human
beings and various fish and animals.

The actual risk of these fungal poisons in our food supply
might be higher than we think. Literally any whole grain or
nut, if not handled properly during production and storage, may
lead to mold growth and, therefore, mycotoxin production.
Besides *aflatoxins*, food scientists are also concerned with
ochratoxin, which causes kidney function disorders. It is
produced by Aspergillus mold found commonly in soil and
commodities like grains, nuts, beans, coffee, fruits, and tobacco; *patulin*, which is mutagenic and carcinogenic as well as
acutely toxic, comes from *Penicillium* mold found commonly in
soil and many fruits including apples (apple cider has been
implicated several times) and even dairy products and meats;

zearalenone, which has been implicated in estrogenic disorders, is a byproduct of a *Fusarium* mold which is very common in grains, corns, and even tomato plants.

There is no doubt that *aflatoxin* receives and deserves the most attention from the government agencies and the food industry. This is because of its common occurrence (especially in ground nuts) and its carcinogenicity. Once this mold poison is in a product, it is very difficult to remove without destroying the product. Even very high temperatures, as in roasting, would only reduce its level slightly. Basically, the maximum allowable level of *aflatoxin* in agriculture is 15 ppb (parts per billion), which is about as far down as scientists can go in detecting the presence of this toxin.

I will never forget when I began working in the food industry. I was paid to crawl inside hot, stuffy boxcars to sample peanuts for *aflatoxin*. And I do mean SAMPLE! Sometimes I had to take up to 48 one-pound samples per lot. You see, out of a bag of peanuts, there may only be a few contaminated nuts, and I really have to make sure that a statistically valid number and size of samples were taken. Then I would mix and grind 48 pounds and take a sample for testing. Can scientists guarantee 100% *aflatoxin*-free nut products by testing? Not really. Unless I used 100% of the peanuts for testing, I would never guarantee a 100% non-toxic product. Obviously, this is not practical!

As the good doctors are now saying, prevention is the key to everything. To minimize *aflatoxin* contamination, we relied on very tight controls during all stages of the production of grains and nuts. This included proper agricultural practices to ensure dry conditions in the field and minimize mechanical damage to the kernel as well as proper storage conditions after harvest. Climate obviously played a big role during this whole process. Most importantly, communication at all levels was essential so that each player along the line knew what to observe in the product. Laboratory testing was only the last line of defense.

Are food products in the market safe from mycotoxins? I would say a qualified "yes." The safety record thus far has been very good. Will anyone guarantee it? Absolutely not. Peanut butter, as well as roasted nut products on the market from reputable suppliers, are quite safe from *aflatoxin* because every batch is usually tested either at the raw ingredient or finished product stage, and often at both stages. If you buy nut products, especially peanut butter, from a small supplier, make sure that the supplier knows what he or she is doing. Shriveled and discolored nut kernels as well as cracked kernels should be avoided.

Grain testing is not done as vigilantly as nut product testing. Although the risk for mycotoxin in grains is smaller than in nut products and the safety record has been good, we should never let down our guards. When dealing with grains, use the same precaution as for nut products. You can never be too careful when it's your own health that you are dealing with. Like Doug says, "Your health matters!"

Inflammatory Bowel Disease and Fungus

by David A. Holland, M.D.

Crohn's disease and ulcerative colitis, although distinguished
by well-known characteristics, are collectively known as
inflammatory bowel diseases (IBD) in the medical arena.
IBD is characterized by a host of symptoms such as diarrhea,
abdominal cramps, rectal bleeding, weight loss, fever, and a
host of extra-intestinal symptoms, including disorders of the
eyes, liver, gallbladder, muscles and joints, kidneys, and skin.
(*Journal of Musculoskeletal Medicine.* Nov. 1996. Pp 28-34.)
Treatment is usually focused on relief of symptoms with anti-
inflammatory drugs or surgery.

The cause of IBD remains unknown. With all of our advances
in medicine, why do the causes of so many diseases remain
unknown?

Some have implicated a viral etiology to IBD. In the medical
journal *The Lancet* (1996. 348:315-317), Dr. Wakefield and
colleagues found that three of four offspring in mothers that
had measles during pregnancy developed severe Crohn's later
in life. Of note is that recurrent antibiotic-resistant pneumonia
preceded the Crohn's in every case.

Others have found carbohydrates to be a possible culprit. Two
of three worldwide studies found the average intake of carbo-

35

hydrates (including bread, potatoes, and refined sugars) to be much greater in those who developed IBD than in those who did not (Heaton, K. W. *Inflammatory Bowel Diseases*. Allan, R.N., Keighley, M.R.B., Alexander-Williams, J., and Hawkins, C.F. [Eds.]. Churchill Livingstone, New York. 1990.).

In her book *Breaking the Vicious Cycle*, Elaine Gottschall describes the cycle of intestinal mucosal injury, impaired digestion, malabsorption, bacterial overgrowth, and increase in bacterial by-products and mucous production which lead back to intestinal mucosal injury. We all know that antibiotics can alter the normal intestinal flora or bacteria. These bacteria usually keep in check the relatively small amount of existing yeast in the intestines. However, when antibiotics are taken for various purposes (and you can bet those kids in Dr. Wakefield's study were given plenty of antibiotics!), the normal protective bacteria are eliminated, and yeast growth goes unchecked. The resulting effects range from "mild diarrhea to severe *colitis*, or *systemic fungal* or bacterial dissemination" (Saadia, Roger and Lipman, Jeffrey. "Antibiotics and the gut". *European Journal of Surgery*. 1996. Suppl. 576:39-41). In Chapter 2, you read about the link between arthritis and fungus. When fungi become systemic from gut inflammation and the overuse of antibiotics, you can see how the whole body becomes involved in what doctors refer to as "gut diseases."

Others have directly implicated the role of yeast in Crohn's disease. Researchers with the World Health Organization (WHO) have found that people with Crohn's often have *aflatoxin*, a fungal poison (refer to Patrick Kwan's article), in their blood. Barclay, G. R., et. al. (*Scandinavian Journal of Gastroenterology*. 1992. 27:196-200) found that disease activity in patients with Crohn's was lower while they followed a yeast-free diet, specifically avoiding baker's and brewer's yeasts.

Over and over we have had patients with symptoms of IBD who have experienced incredible improvement once they followed a yeast free, low carbohydrate diet. We have been a little more aggressive, though, and have added antifungal medicines like Nystatin which seem to speed up the improvement by inhibiting any further fungal growth.

Chapter 13 of *Principles and Practice of Clinical Mycology* (Kibbler, C. C., et. al [Ed.]. 1996. John Wiley & Sons, Ltd., West Sussex, England.) deals entirely with fungal infections in the gut. They describe how *Blastomyces dermatitidis*, a fungus, can produce granulomatous lesions in the intestines. Interestingly, this type of lesion has also been seen in patients with Crohn's disease. Another fungus called *Histoplasma* produced intestinal disease with symptoms such as diarrhea, weight loss, fever, and abdominal pain – sound familiar? The common lesions seen in the gut with this infection were "masses or ulcers mimicking inflammatory bowel disease or carcinoma." The authors concluded that *histoplasmosis* should be a serious consideration in an immunocompromised patient with signs and symptoms of IBD. Now back to the big word "immunocompromised," which means a weak immune system. We strongly disagree that you must have cancer or AIDS or be on chemotherapy to have a weakened immune system. Just smell the air on your way to work or look at our standard American diet (SAD). Could these be impeding our immune systems? Anyone who has been diagnosed with ulcerative colitis or Crohn's disease knows the misery these diseases can cause. Given the alternatives for treatment, we think it would be worth a trial on a good antifungal program that includes diet, antifungals, and desensitization to the fungi.

Gut Fungi and the Diseases They Mimic:
Is It Crohn's or Is It Fungus?

by Doug A. Kaufmann

So you've just been diagnosed with one of the many intestinal disorders! Well, before you take another anti-inflammatory pill or consider surgery, you absolutely must know that there is a chance that the medical community may be misdiagnosing many gut diseases.

In 1983, the *New England Journal of Medicine* published a correspondence letter from four doctors at the University of Tennessee Center for the Health Sciences. These doctors had learned that psoriasis (a skin condition that dermatologists do not know the cause of) and Crohn's disease (an intestinal disease that gastroenterologists do not know the cause of) may both be caused by yeast. Imagine that! One of the doctors, E. William Rosenberg, M.D., had previously discovered serendipitously that while treating skin diseases with the antifungal drug Nystatin, several of the patients also had their Crohn's disease symptoms reverse. The doctors stated, "We suspect, therefore, that gut yeast may have a role in some instances of psoriasis." And the same with Crohn's disease! How right they are, but why have fourteen years gone by without making this important announcement?

Long before 1983, I learned that the Tennessee doctor's statement above was absolutely true and I set out to reverse these terrible diseases. Although I have been successful in doing this, I have been unsuccessful in teaching doctors about this incredible discovery. But why should I even have to try? Why aren't gastroenterologists receiving the life saving information that many gut diseases are really just fungal diseases in disguise? Could the answer be associated with the money trail?

Recently, I was invited to lecture to a group of Crohn's and colitis sufferers at a local hospital. Just before I was introduced, the man in charge handed me a brochure dispensed by all chapters of the Crohn's & Colitis Foundation of America (CCFA). It was entitled, "Questions and Answers about Diet & Nutrition." To make a long story short, this brochure stated very clearly that there was no special diet for these diseases and no foods worsened the symptoms. And who do you suppose would have produced this brochure? The very industry that has a vested financial interest in keeping people with intestinal diseases on medicines! This brochure was produced by a grant from Solvay Pharmaceuticals, the makers of Rowasa, rectal suppositories for intestinal diseases!

A Personal Story of Healing

A Testimonial
by F. G., Fort Worth, Texas

I moved to Texas in November 1982, and all was well with my health until about two years later (1984) when I started developing allergies. These allergies got to the point where I started getting sinus infections almost monthly. Every month I would go back to the doctor and get another round of antibiotics for these infections.

After about a year of this, I went to see a specialist and he discovered polyps in my sinuses. Although he surgically removed them, my sinus infections persisted. Once again, I found myself going to the doctor for more antibiotics. I finally went to an allergist and started getting desensitizing shots and prescriptions for decongestants, antihistamines, and topical nasal steroids. This did not help with my chronic sinus infections, so he offered me, you guessed it, antibiotics!

During one of my infections, I didn't feel like eating much of anything for three days. No one had told me that when you take the combination of antihistamines, decongestants, and antibiotics, you should always eat – I learned the hard way. After sitting at my desk for five hours, I began to get light-headed and my heart started racing. This put me in the emergency room and I spent three days in a cardiac care unit.

Luckily, I didn't have a heart attack, but I went through all of the testing, treadmill, stress thallium, echo cardiogram, and finally the cardiac catheter. Although my heart checked out fine, I continued to feel terrible.

For several years after that, I continued on the same routine with regard to my health: chronic sinus infections and antibiotics. This process would continue until 1993 when I discovered blood in my stools. After numerous trips to my primary care physician, I was finally sent to a specialist. They determined I had "antibiotic colitis." They prescribed cheese and yogurt. For six months my symptoms cleared and then they began again. Again, I returned to my primary care doctor numerous times and again he referred me to another specialist. I waited three weeks for an appointment. During this time, I really thought I was dying! Now chills, fever, and diarrhea were everyday occurrences. The specialist did a colonoscopy and I was diagnosed with ulcerative colitis. He prescribed Prednisone and sulfasalazine to help control the symptoms. This initiated a long roller coaster ride, my health suffered and my symptoms returned with a vengeance.

In November of 1995 I was hospitalized for a week because of dehydration, loss of blood, and severe abdominal pain. I had heard of a person who owned a health food store and later learned that they could recommend some natural products that might help me with my condition. The same day the hospital released me, I went to the health food store. There I was loaded up with more than one hundred and fifty dollars worth of natural products. After reading all of the directions, I was supposed to take approximately 40 pills per day at various times and drink three different kinds of herbal concoctions. I attempted to stay on this program, but it caused my symptoms to worsen.

The following month I was back in the hospital for another week. The doctor notified me that if my condition did not improve within a few days, he would recommend surgical removal of my colon. The next day, the surgeon who was slated to do the surgery came into my room and detailed the surgical procedure for me. Fortunately for me, the 200 plus milligrams of Prednisone I was receiving in my IV started to work and I was able to put off the surgery.

At this time, I felt that surgical removal of my colon was inevitable, so I thought it was important for me to talk with others who had had this surgery. I was able to attend a support group meeting for persons with ulcerative colitis and Crohn's disease. This meeting would turn my life around.

The guest speakers at this meeting were Doug Kaufmann and Dr. David Holland. They talked about the effects of antibiotics on the digestive system and of fungus within the colon. I soon realized that there were many similarities with my condition.

The following week I made an appointment to see them. Dr. Holland went over the restrictive diet program with me and prescribed some antifungal medicines that I needed to take. The following day my wife and I began the diet. To be honest, the first three days were almost unbearable, but after that I got used to eating the foods. During the first two weeks I noticed that the abdominal pain that I had lived with for the past three years was completely gone! My stools were completely normal and I felt better than I did before I was diagnosed with ulcerative colitis. An added benefit to this diet was that I have taken off four inches from my waist, my blood pressure went down considerably, and my sinuses are clear. I can't pretend to completely understand this process, but I cannot argue with the results. I can thank Doug and Dr. Holland for giving me a normal life again!

Treating an "Incurable" Disease

A Testimonial
by Russ J.

I was first diagnosed with Crohn's disease at the age of 14, a little over 20 years ago. Since then, my primary symptoms have been diarrhea and anal fistulas. I have been on and off a variety of medications: Prednisone, Azulfidine, Asacol, Rowasa, Flagyl, and Cipro. I have had a total of six surgeries, which altogether removed about two-thirds of my colon or large intestine. Many of these things helped for a period of months or even years, but then my symptoms began to reappear or even worsen. Sometimes my fistulas got so painful that I began carrying a "fanny cushion" (made for hemorrhoid sufferers) with me everywhere I went and I took daily sitz baths.

At the beginning of 1996, I first heard about the Specific Carbohydrate Diet (SC). On the internet, I read testimonials of people who had been cured using the diet. My wife and I read a book that explained a low carbohydrate diet in detail and it gave many good recipes. I subscribed to a free, electronic mail Specific Carbohydrate Diet discussion/support group (now at sed@filmgraphics.com). This proved to be a great source of encouragement, information, and additional recipes.

In March 1996, my wife and I started the SC Diet. I began to see good results within a few days. After about ten days on the diet, I found myself having four to six bowel movements per day rather than the 10 to 12 I had previously had. Over the next few months I saw continued progress. I could often make it through a nine hour workday without having to "go." Prior to this diet, I went three to five times during the workday. Eventually my fistulas cleared up enough that I was able to get off both Flagyl and Cipro, which had been specifically prescribed to treat them. My wife's seasonal allergy symptoms seemed to get much better. This diet was really working great!

However, after ten months on the diet, I still had one persistent anal fistula and was still not having "normal" bowel movements. I had seemed to reach a plateau. I was much better than before the diet, but was frustrated that I saw little, if any, additional progress. I started listening to Doug Kaufmann on the radio, and he discussed the role of candida (a type of yeast) in many diseases, including Crohn's disease. Doug and David Holland, M.D., were going to discuss this correlation at a local meeting of a CCFA (Crohn's and Colitis Foundation of America) support group. I went and was impressed with what I heard. I made an appointment with them at Nutrition Resources the following week.

For two weeks they put me on a slightly stricter diet, which they refer to as an initial phase diet. Dr. Holland prescribed Nystatin, an antifungal drug, and they told me to begin taking daily doses of psyllium hulls. This is a source of non-digestible fiber available at health food stores. Several of the 100+ members of the SC Diet e-mail had suggested the same things. As I had been warned, my diarrhea got slightly worse for the first few days on the program as yeast in my system began to "die off." By day ten on their program, I had the first normal bowel movement I'd had in several years!

Since then I have been able to reduce by 1/3 the dosage of Asacol (an anti-inflammatory drug) that I have been on for 18 months. A week ago, Dr. Holland prescribed Diflucan, a systemic antifungal drug, which we hope will help my one persistent fistula. Apparently, Nystatin does not get into the blood stream, so it might be unable to reach the fistula. Again, I experienced some yeast die-off upon starting Diflucan, but that reaction seems to have subsided now. I am looking forward to seeing continued progress.

Many people in the medical community see Crohn's disease as an incurable disease that remains undaunted by diet. My experience seems to prove otherwise. I thank God for leading me to the help that I needed.

Chapter Four

Relating Fungus to Respiration

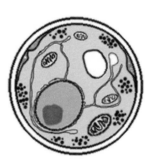

Respiratory Disorders and Fungus

by Doug A. Kaufmann

In our lives there can be nothing more fearful than the inability to breathe. Having one's airway constricted so tightly that suffocation ensues is frightening. Many believe that Jesus suffocated on the cross. This was the price He paid for our sins. Why must millions of Americans suffer so terrible a fate every day? And why do Americans suffer more than any other people in the world with this affliction? The answer may amaze you!

I read with awe and disbelief the May 1997 issue of *Life* magazine. The cover is entirely dedicated to respiratory distress. But the cover also sold a ray of hope to readers. It said, "If you are one of the 50 million Americans with allergies or asthma, now you can take control of your life." The hope they offered centered on "new discoveries, smarter drugs, and breakthrough therapies." All of this, of course, we've been hearing for the past 50 years. Hmmm, now wait a minute! 50 years ago antibiotics were first introduced to American children! It just couldn't be that simple, could it? Because doctors and researchers would have already figured that one out! Read on.

The *Life* magazine article opened with the most unbelievable two sentences I have ever read. Let me quote them for you:

"Jeremiah Jager, four, loves blue. He drinks blue soda pop, picks the blue marshmallows out of his Magic Star cereal, and grabs the blue crayon." Do you think even *one* physician examining Jeremiah saw a link between his asthma and the dangerous blue dyes in the food he eats? My guess would be "no!"

In their defense, medical doctors have licenses that preclude them from acknowledging anything medical except what they learned in medical school. This, despite their own Hippocratic oath which recites, "I will use dietetic measures whenever possible." Should a physician question, for example, that the antibiotics previously used on Jeremiah might initiate or exacerbate his asthma, he would stand a chance of being reprimanded by the medical board in his state. Drug companies pay a great deal of money to medical schools and medical researchers. A fiduciary relationship exists between the senior medical staff and the providers of income streams. So, for a physician to even question that those providing money might in any way be involved in keeping Americans sick and in hospitals is un-American and unthinkable! And don't you even *think* of implicating chemical dyes in respiratory diseases. Remember that drugs are chemicals and chemical companies make blue dyes.

If I were a "fungally informed" physician, the first thing I would do is to tell Jeremiah's parents to immediately change his favorite color to orange. Get him off of the blue food he is eating and begin juicing with carrot juice daily. You see, the enzymes, beta-carotene, and vitamin A liberated from organic carrots alone could help his breathing condition. In 1988, the *Journal of Microbiology* published a paper which confirmed that carrots have an ingredient that inhibited candida organisms by damaging its cell membrane. Candida albicans is likely the yeast that Jeremiah has harbored in his lungs for many years following antibiotic use. The yeast (fungus) condition that mimics asthma is called *bronchial pulmonary candidiasis.*

I would encourage Jeremiah's parents to get a prescription from their doctor for Nystatin suspension 100,000/ml and have Jeremiah take this harmless soil-based antifungal medicine following the morning meal and the evening meal. I would educate the Jagers, including Jeremiah, that if a fungus has gained access to his lungs, it is living and it is parasitic (it requires food from Jeremiah's diet). I would inform them that certain foods like soda pop and cereals feed the fungus and make it branch out even more, possibly infecting other tissues than just his lungs at some later time in his life. Doctors who understand these dangerous fungi have reported their presence in *every tissue in the human body,* and many are only found at autopsy, when it is too late to treat them.

What upset me more than the content of this *Life* magazine article was the fact that I smelled a skunk! The article appeared to me to be nothing more than a sales pitch to get more unfortunate pediatric recruits for the National Jewish Medical and Research Center in Denver. Don't get me wrong, I'm certain there are wonderful medical people involved with this prestigious center. But I also know that each needs a paycheck. And just how do they get this paycheck? Jeremiah's insurance company paid $17,000 for a ten day visit! Jeremiah came in with asthma and he went home ten days later with asthma and it only cost $17,000! Medical mediocrity at its best!

Do you think it would have worked for this hospital to have a physician sit down for two hours with the Jagers and to change Jeremiah's diet and to inquire as to whether the asthma initiated after a round of antibiotics? The question is, *worked for whom*? Yes, it would have likely worked for the Jagers. No, it wouldn't have worked for the hospital. And something I will never understand is why in the world powerful insurance giants allow their money to be flushed into the medical institutions the way they do. I am relatively certain that those in power in these insurance companies really do believe that they are doing the right thing. And if they want to throw away their money, far be it from me to challenge such illogical behavior. But when it's all gone, watch them crawl into health food stores for relief of the stress they've self-imposed. So, Jeremiah suffers, insurance companies waste money, and hospitals and their staffs keep the patients flowing. Is it any wonder that we in America continue to suffer?

Is It Asthma or Is It Fungus?

by David A. Holland, M. D.

Harrison's Principles of Internal Medicine, 12th Edition, defines asthma this way: "A disease of the airways that is character-ized by increased responsiveness of the tracheobronchial tree to a multiplicity of stimuli … manifested physiologically by a widespread narrowing of the air passages, which may be relieved spontaneously or as a result of therapy, and clinically by paroxysms of dypsnea, cough, and wheezing. It is an episodic disease, acute exacerbations being interspersed with symptom-free periods."

Is it possible to make something so complicated that we miss the simplicity of it? As with other diseases we have previously covered in *The Fungazette*, the cause of asthma is often un-known. With a few cases we are able to pinpoint the cause, whether it is a chemical that is inhaled, causing lung damage, or an environmental dust like cement that can irritate the bronchial linings in the lungs and trigger wheezing and bron-chial spasms in the worker, or victim. Once again, we will be looking at the role of fungus in this disease. We may as well include allergies, also known as allergic rhinitis, along with asthma in this discussion.

Often patients have both asthma and allergies, and the allergies can sometimes trigger the asthma or simply cause the daily misery of sniffles and congestion that you know if you are unfortunate enough to have experienced allergies. We hope to offer some simplicity to a disease that is approached with so much complexity.

I recently reviewed an overview of asthma prepared by the pharmaceutical company Glaxo Wellcome, Inc., entitled, *Asthma Market Overview*. So, asthma is a market. A source of millions of dollars in profits. I guess that's OK; after all, we all have the opportunity to make a profit in this country. It is the people with asthma who fail to take an interest in their health who will continue to contribute to this market. Obviously, you are not one of these people. You have decided to stop the money trail by taking an interest and learning more about your particular condition. Whether this information helps you or not, we deeply appreciate the effort you are making to recapture your health. Let's look at some of the figures mentioned in this asthma report:

"An estimated 15 million Americans suffer from asthma, including 4.8 million children and adolescents."
(CDC. *Asthma mortality and hospitalization among children and young adults – U.S.* 1980-1993. MMWR)

"The prevalence of asthma is increasing substantially (38% over the past decade)."
(CDC. *Asthma – U.S. 1980-1990*. MMWR. 1992:41:733-735).

I wonder if 38% more antibiotics have been used over the last ten years.

"The total estimated cost of asthma in 1990 was $6.2 billion,
up 38% from 1985."

(Weiss, K. B., Gergen, P. J., Hodgson, T. A.
" An economic evaluation of asthma in the United States. "
New England Journal of Medicine. 1992. 326:862-866).

Based on these figures, whoever helps people substantially
with their asthma is going to make a lot of money by taking the
market share and upsetting the pharmaceutical companies at the
same time! Overall though, they will be contributing to
significant savings in both therapy and lives. Often we forget
that there is human life behind all of these figures.

And then there was the *Life* magazine issue that Doug mentioned in his article "Respiratory Disorders and Fungus."
There are two references in this article that I would like to
expound on. First of all, it is widely known that sugar has the
ability to depress the immune system. Anyone with a potentially fatal illness (around 5,200 people still die of asthma each
year) should not be gambling with blue soda pop and Magic
Star cereal. Cane sugar is a notoriously moldy food, and when
consumed is able to introduce molds and their toxins directly
into the human body. Speaking of mold, the article also refers
to another asthmatic child named Nathan: "Eight year old
Nathan Skinner's former home tests positive for mold." Some
mold growing in homes has been known to cause respiratory
diseases and even bleeding from the lungs. Based on this
observation my question might be: should Nathan be moved out
of the moldy house or simply be prescribed more medicines to
reduce the potentially toxic effect of the mold on his respiratory
system?

57

An article by Kauffman, H. F., et. al. ("Review of fungus-induced asthmatic reactions." *American Journal of Respiratory Critical Care Medicine.* June 1995.) outlines the ability of fungus to not only cause an allergic reaction by simple exposure to the lungs, but also *colonize* the lungs and induce an inflammatory reaction from the infection. How common is this? A different Dr. Kauffman states that, "each year in the U. S. the fungi *Histoplasma capsulatum, Blastomyces dermatitidis,* and *Coccidioides immitis* cause more pulmonary infections than bacteria." (Kauffman, Carol A., M.D. "Nonresolving pneumonia: Is endemic mycoses to blame?" *The Journal of Respiratory Diseases.* Vol. 16. No 11. Nov 1995.) According to C. C. Kibbler, these fungi "routinely infect persons with apparently normal immunity" (*Principles and Practices of Clinical Mycology.* 1996. John Wiley & Sons, Ltd.) Ever notice that the asthma you once had as a child is no longer bothering you as an adult? It is well known that sensitization to fungi is higher in the early years and declines rapidly as we age (Kauffman, H. F., et. al.).

If fungal infections, then, can contribute to asthma and allergies, why not treat asthma, when the cause is unknown, empirically as if a fungus caused it?

In a study on allergic broncho-pulmonary aspergillosis, a fungus-induced condition that can essentially mimic asthma and is a common complication of cystic fibrosis, **100%** (six out of six) of the patients treated with the antifungal drug Sporanox experienced improvement in lung function (Dennis, David W., et. al. Adjunctive Therapy of Allergic Bronchopulmonary

Aspergillosis with Itraconazole. Chest 100; 3:813-819. Sept 1991.). This was a small study done in 1991. No interest in a larger study has occurred so far.

Another so-called "cause" of asthma, you may have been told, is reflux. That is, reflux of acid from the stomach up the esophagus and back down into the lungs, causing irritation of the lining of the bronchioles. Can this really be fungus as well? You guessed it – the most common cause of *Candida albicans* bronchopneumonia is from aspiration of oral secretions. Everybody aspirates a small amount of either oral secretions or stomach fluids at night while sleeping. If large amounts of yeast can cause pneumonia in a debilitated person, can it "just" cause asthma in a normal person? The question would be, is the acid causing the lung irritation, or is it the yeast that is sneaking in along with the fluids? And if it is the acid, what is causing it to reflux in the first place? We should not even have to answer that question!

We once saw a prominent man who had asthma and was spending upwards of $600 a month on asthma medications. He lived in a small town in Texas and, because of his frequent trips to the pharmacy, he had become good friends with the pharmacist.

In desperation and in light of not seeing any improvement after much time, he sought our help. We advised a particular diet known to starve fungi (vital to the program), a few supplements, and empirically, like the above study did, prescribed antifungal medications. The results were no less than dramatic.

He lost weight, looked younger because of that, and was able to shed all of his asthma medication. The only dissatisfied party was the pharmacist, who no longer returned his phone calls.

Bronchial Politics: How and Why "Asthmaphobia" was Created

by Doug A. Kaufmann

Why did two of the most established magazines in the United States, *Life* and *Newsweek,* devote their entire cover page to asthma in May of 1997? Could this be a public relations move on the part of the American Lung Association (ALA)? And just who are these folks that dedicate their lives to the well being of American lungs? Charities are often the public relations entities for the medical communities that they represent. According to the book *Unhealthy Charities,* you'd be surprised at who these "charities" are charitable to. About 13 years ago, one of my employees lost her father to cancer. My worst nightmare came true. I received a letter from her requesting that in lieu of flowers I make a "charitable contribution" to the American Cancer Society (ACS). Call it what you may, to this day I feel that my donation made a Porsche payment for a "cancer expert" affiliated with the ACS. Why is the grieving and bereavement process made socially acceptable in America only if a donation is made to a charity?

I, for one, will never ever donate another dime to a charity. Less than five percent (5%) of the funds raised by the ALA for "urgent need" research actually goes to any research at all! The other 95% apparently covers costs, including payroll. According to the above referenced book, the ALA is a marketing wing for the respiratory organizations, purportedly including doctors, who treat lung problems. So why all the PR on asthma? They're just doing their job. The more frightened parents they recruit into one of these hospitals, the more awareness is generated. Then it's just a matter of educating the parents on the wonderful job that the hospitals did to save their children's lives. Seemingly, a donation to the very charity that saved their child's life and then educated them on the complexity of breathing would be fitting. It's all marketing, kids!

So why should charitable money be invested in trying to figure out what causes respiratory diseases? Because medical institutions only make money when we're in them! It is my opinion that in their effort to keep us ignorant, they are making a few sloppy mistakes. The *Newsweek* article on asthma, for example, stated that "with the rise in vaccines and antibiotics, people in developed countries have experienced fewer serious childhood infections than ever before." Yet a survey published in *The Journal of the American Medical Association* reported that children receiving the pertussis vaccine were six times more likely to develop asthma than those not receiving the vaccination. And one only needs to review medical mycology to know that antibiotics can actually cause asthma. If it were true that our medical breakthroughs, i.e., antibiotics and vaccines, had reduced the number of asthma occurrences in America (certainly a "developed country"), how might you explain the fact that asthma rates have dramatically increased in every age group since 1982?

I believe that what irritates me most is the fact that the medical associations via their promotional and purportedly "non-profit" associations, seem to be preying on children. That is apparently their "target market." The mentality seems to be, "It's done with cigarettes, why not with asthma?" Each of the magazines mentioned above has small, helpless children on the cover.

Have you been watching the news or reading the newspapers lately? It seems that we have yet another medical epidemic on our hands. This one is called diabetes. It is now called the "hidden killer," because many of us have it and don't know it. And if we don't get to a doctor, we may die! Well, I predict that if this ad campaign for asthma doesn't increase hospital revenues enough, very soon asthma and other respiratory diseases will be billed as "toxic time bombs" ticking away in our children. And all of this is done in such a way as to make you feel that their concern is genuine. Indeed, I've long felt that most medical people have very high integrity, and remember: they are not to blame. But I am concerned about the integrity of those who have found that the secret to making money in medicine is through confusion and deception...scare tactics, if you will. Simply put, there are many to whom you are worth considerably more sick than when you are well. Your job is to use your head when consuming medical products or services.

I would never allow any one diagnosis to dictate my next move with my children. First, I'd see a medical doctor, followed by a health food store owner, followed by a chiropractor, followed by a nurse, and lastly a good (the good part is sometimes the most difficult) nutritional expert. I would never be fooled into believing that credentials in lieu of experience "made" the health care provider. Every day thousands of children are prescribed medicines for asthma by people with wonderful credentials; but I have known health food store owners who have amassed far safer and more logical treatment plans than chiefs of medical departments. Next, I'd take all of the knowledge that each person provided and I'd find someone I trust to help me with my decision. Knowing all of this should allow you, and your child, to breathe easier – and without a $17,000 bill.

A Personal Story of Healing

A Testimonial
by MFE, Plano, Texas

After I first met Doug Kaufmann, I finally began to see the light at the end of the tunnel. I cannot believe how much better I feel. Thanks to him, I have a life again. My only regret is not having met him earlier in my life and been given the ability to take charge of my life and my health.

Looking back over my medical history makes me realize just how long I suffered from Candida albicans. Over the years I was misdiagnosed by so many medical doctors and professionals that it is ridiculous. I realize now they treated the symptoms of my disease and not the problem, often masking the real problems with drugs. My whole way of thinking has changed so drastically that I will never trust my health in their hands again!

Back in 1972 I was diagnosed with asthma. I had always thought of asthma as a childhood disease, yet I was 16 years old. I was given expensive pulmonary function tests to measure and regulate the function of my lungs. I was treated with drugs, bronchial inhalers, and strong steroids.

From this point forward, I found myself shifting from one health crisis to another, never realizing until now that it was all connected to a fungus in my lungs. While my health continued to fail, the most dangerous focal point was always my asthma and lungs. Anytime I got the slightest cold or flu, I was prescribed a round of antibiotics to eliminate any further accumulation of fluids or germs in my lungs.

Around 1973 to '74, I began taking birth control pills to help regulate my menstrual periods and eliminate the painful abdominal cramping that accompanied them. I was also given strong pain medicine for the cramping. Today, I do not even need Tylenol. My asthma began requiring additional medical attention and stronger doses of the already prescribed medication.

In 1978, my medical doctor informed me that I would never live to be 40 years old because of my severe asthma.

In 1981, I married and on my honeymoon I got diarrhea that lasted four to five months. As I was euphoric, I passed this malady off to eating rich foods and making lifestyle adjustments. Again, medical doctors gave me enough drugs to stop the diarrhea to the point of constipation. No medical tests were run.

At this point in my life, I was a young professional woman at a high point in my career. I traveled, never exercised, and drank heavily – eating whenever I could. I paid little attention to any damage incurred and had my doctor's phone number memorized. He had even given me his private number for convenience reasons in case of emergency, as he considered me a regular patient with chronic asthma problems and the clock was ticking! He had already told me that I did not have long to live.

From this point, I was always the first one to have a cold, infectious bronchitis, and the flu. All I ever had to do was call my doctor who happily treated me over the phone, convincing me I needed a prescription of antibiotics to clear up any chest congestion, which would eliminate further complications. It would be true to say that I relied on my doctor heavily and trusted him to take care of my needs or this cycle would not have continued for as long as it did. I do not mean to blame everything on my doctor, but I was brought up to find a good doctor and then trust in him completely for all of my health needs. I even depended on him for referrals to other physicians when needed.

In 1983, I quit taking the birth control pills and became pregnant. During this period of time, I seemed to be relatively healthy. It was great! Other than some morning sickness during my first trimester, I enjoyed my pregnancy. Although I was big, I felt beautiful and very healthy. Following a normal vaginal delivery and nine months of nursing, I unfortunately resumed taking the birth control pills.

In 1986, I began to have chronic fungal problems under my toenails and was referred to a general surgeon for laser surgery. While this surgery was considered minor, the doctor stated that he had never seen anything like this before and he took many pictures in amazement. I required several additional surgeries (at least three) as the fungal warts kept returning with a vengeance. After each surgery, I was given antibiotics and pain medication.

Also during this time, I was in a severe car accident resulting in spinal fusion surgery along with more pain medications, muscle relaxers, and antibiotics for infection.

In 1992, thrush symptoms began in my mouth. The center of my tongue was white and had a film or coating on it while the sides were swollen, cracked, and had sensitive white patches. I also had diarrhea. My trusted physician diagnosed me as having eaten too much cinnamon candy and placed me on a bland diet for two weeks.

In 1993, my periods began to become a bother again, although I was on birth control and pain medication. I was given stronger pain mediation and a series of sympathetic handshakes. Finally, I was referred to numerous doctors for various treatments before being diagnosed with endometriosis. I did not want a hysterectomy, which was the "normal" procedure to correct this problem. Three of four doctors I consulted wanted my permission for a total hysterectomy surgical procedure based on my symptoms alone. The fourth doctor agreed to an exploratory procedure, based on my apparent apprehension, before performing a hysterectomy. The results of this exploratory procedure were overwhelming! I had the insides of a newborn baby – pretty and pink.

My pain continued and the doctor stated that I had pelvic congestion due to lack of satisfactory sex with my husband. He sent me home with a package of birth control pills. He suggested that these pills along with regular sex with my husband would take care of any pain or problems I was having.

In 1994, I began to develop another series of unidentifiable symptoms diagnosed as depression. At this time, the phrase "all in your head" began to take on a new meaning. I consulted numerous medical professionals and patience was wearing thin at my house. Medical doctors placed me on anti-depression therapy and further acknowledged the previous diagnosis of "it's all in your head." In other words, they had no clue as to what was wrong with me or what to do about it, so I must be crazy.

In 1995, I sustained a minor car accident injury resulting in an accumulation (later discovered) of mold and mildew in the trunk of my car. At this point, my health deteriorated to the "point of no return." Remembering that several years earlier my "trusted physician" had predicted that I would not live to be 40 years old, I truly believed that his prediction was finally coming true. I was dying.

Although only 39 years old, I found myself buying, planning, and paying for my own funeral. My husband took us on a fabulous trip for our fifteenth wedding anniversary. I was very sick for the entire trip. I could not keep food in my stomach for more than 15 minutes and found it embarrassing to eat. This was in May of 1996. To add to my frustration, during this time my husband lost his job and we had no medical insurance.

Upon arriving home, my severe asthma and diarrhea were horrible. The medical professionals advised me to drink Pepto Bismol daily and take prescriptive medicine to relieve the diarrhea. To their amazement, nothing worked – not even the strongest medication they prescribed. I use the term "medical professionals" because I went to several, none of whom could help me. They ran all kinds of tests, took blood and stool samples, and found absolutely nothing wrong with me. I found it more frustrating than they did, probably because they had my money for their services yet each looked at me with skepticism, whispers, and frowns.

After another run-around with the medical professionals, God blessed me and I found Nutrition Resources. I was a total mess. My body could not hold food for more than fifteen minutes. I could not sleep, I cried all the time, was irrational and hard to get along with. I am certain that my husband would agree with this statement. When asked, "How do you feel?" I had mixed emotions. I felt sorry for anyone who loved or cared for me. I had been an emotional roller coaster basket case for many years and had never known why. I had been irrational, hot tempered, and sick without reason time after time.

Someone once said, "Smile, smile, things are not too bad." I had forgotten how to smile. When asked, "What do you do for fun?" I really had to think: fun – what is that? Fun was a privilege I had not enjoyed for so long I had forgotten what it was. I can not even believe that my husband still found me attractive. Most men would have left me a long time ago.

I had prayed to God to give wisdom to the doctors who tried to help me, and I found Doug. My girlfriend had tried to persuade me to call him for quite a while. However, I was skeptical of anyone but a medical doctor. Looking back, I now feel like such a fool. Immediately, Doug identified my problem and taught me that what I had been eating was actually causing my health problems. I just couldn't believe it!

Within two weeks, my diarrhea was completely gone and I began a long journey of healing. The road certainly has been filled with bumps full of skepticism and criticism – especially to those who claim to love me the most. I began to experience what Doug referred to as "Herxheimer's reaction," more commonly known as the "die-off" of fungus.

Once again, I felt as if I was dying. My hands were shaky, my vision was blurred, my ears were ringing, I experienced numbness in my hands and legs, I was depressed, disoriented, and confused. Extremely fatigued, my severe headaches persisted, my hair began to fall out, and I cried most of the time. I dropped out of college for lack of concentration skills, and I felt worthless. My complexion took on a pasty white appearance and those around me constantly stared with horror on their faces. Numerous times I was told that I should find another doctor or seek another opinion. Thank God I did not. I stuck it out and now those problems are behind me. I really feel that Doug saved my life or at least gave me a life back. I am forever grateful for him and his staff.

Dr. Holland became a great source of support and I relied on his medical guidance coupled with their treatment plan for recovery. On several occasions, I have slipped off the diet and found myself in respiratory failure needing immediate attention. Help was only a phone call away. I cannot thank you all enough.

Chapter Five

Relating Fungus to
Brain Disorders and Mental Health

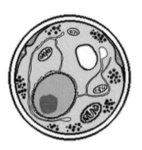

Fungal Related Brain Disorders

by Doug A. Kaufmann

While working with Dr. Everett Hughes in USC Medical School, I collaborated on a research paper that dealt with attention deficit disorders and its link to diet. The paper concluded that, indeed, diet was a factor in many cases of ADD. This information and years of study piqued my interest in abnormal brain reactions caused by food and fungi.

Many years ago *Life* magazine presented a visual exploration of the intricate areas of the brain. This issue went where no other issue, or magazine for that matter, had ever gone: literally inside the human brain. Once inside this issue, readers discovered that although the visuals were excellent and intriguing, scientists still knew little about what this mass actually did.

This information void still exists today. Yes, we know more than we did in 1960, but considering that this organ governs our thoughts, our understandings, and our intellect, it is surprising that 20th century medicine knows so little about the brain's interactions with other parts of our body, let alone our nervous system.

The research possibilities are limitless when dealing with the brain and the nervous system. And there are very few "knowns." In lieu of understanding how the brain works, let's evaluate how the brain might react to extraneous factors ... say, fungal organisms. The scientific literature speaks about *meningeal* fungi. The meninges are the three coatings of the brain and the spinal cord. Since it is well documented that fungi can enter the blood stream, it is logical that these fungi can impregnate virtually any tissues in the body, including the meningeal tissues. In 1995, a medical textbook entitled *Medical Mycology* devoted an entire chapter to fungal meningitis. The "-itis" on the end of that word indicates an inflammation of the meninges. And just what caused the meninges to swell? Absolutely right – fungus!

I am probably guilty of being too logical when it comes to long words and medical jargon, but it has always seemed to me that if yeast can make bread swell, it can certainly make organs like the brain and its billions of connected cells (people) swell, also. Hence, *Medical Mycology* is one of many books that implicate fungi in brain swelling. Exactly what happens when the brain and spinal cord tissues swell is yet to be fully understood, but it can not be good! Doesn't cerebral swelling cause some headaches? Since certain areas of the brain control appetite while others control behavior, couldn't swelling impact those two as well?

Researchers have discovered six relatively common fungi that can invade the spinal cord. One, Candida albicans, can cause problems anywhere in the body. Another, Cryptococci, primarily invades the meningeal tissues. Doctors say that people with impaired immune systems generally end up with the most health problems when this happens; but do they really?

Sometimes when people follow a specific program to eradicate fungi from their bodies, their brain symptoms clear up. These are some of the most exciting cases you have ever seen. It is my humble opinion that many people who are relegated to a life of phobias, tears, and antidepressants may really have an underlying fungal root to their cerebral symptoms. There is not a magic pill, diet, or exercise program that will create overnight success. Rather, an all-encompassing program must be initiated. And it can safely be done while continuing on antidepressants.

This area of fungal proliferation is important. It is important to explore the relationship between aberrant behavior and fungus within the brain. The important consideration is whether brain problems are psychological or physiological.

Diet, Dimorphic Fungi, and Depression

by Doug A. Kaufmann

Roses are red, violets are blue,
I'm schizophrenic, and so am I!

~~~

A man walks into a psychiatrist's office with a
large frog on his head. The psychiatrist says,
"My, you seem to have a significant problem."
The frog replies, "Yes, and until I can get this
growth removed from my belly, it's likely to
become more significant!"

~~~

There are no shortages of puns or jokes directed at the mentally
impaired. True depression, however, is no joking matter. Nor,
say the statisticians, is it rare. There are approximately 14
million Americans who suffer from depression (World Book
Encyclopedia). According to a *Newsweek* magazine article
published in 1990, at that time, doctors wrote or renewed about
60,000 Prozac prescriptions monthly (*Newsweek*. March 30,
1990). Just imagine today's count!

All of this data suggests that there are no shortages of depressed people or doctors willing to temporarily erase their
symptoms. When dealing with depression, the question that

continues to perplex medical scientists is: If we are merely erasing symptoms of depression with medication, what are they symptoms of?

I do not believe that depressed people suffer from a deficiency of selective seratonin reuptake inhibitors (SSRI). Yet, Prozac is but one of these medications meant to ease depression – a few hours per pill. There are actually numerous SSRIs and antidepressant medications, all aimed at controlling a symptom. There's that word again: symptom. What is depression a symptom of? Could it be fungus?!

The purpose of this book is to tackle not only physical symptoms of fungal infections but mental symptoms as well, and to educate people about how to recapture the health that most of them once had and that a few have never experienced.

The Fungal Link to Depression

by David A. Holland, M. D.

There is not one of you reading this who has not either experienced depression or known someone who has experienced it. Depression is a normal human emotion; in fact, the lack of depression in certain situations, like the loss of a loved one, can be abnormal. There are different degrees of depression. That which we will be discussing is the degree of depression that is defined as a clinical illness. Just like diabetes, depression is defined by clinical criteria which may not be obvious to the majority of people but have important implications in treatment and in seeking the causes of the depression.

Depression is also a powerful condition: its presence in someone's life can affect decisions they make in their relationships or business decisions that can have dramatic consequences for that person's future. It can also affect one's self esteem, one's value of life, and one's value of health, as well. It can break up marriages and cause job loss, hopelessness, and even suicide. In short, as Doug mentioned, it is no laughing matter.

What this article hopes to suggest is that there may be a link to fungi in many cases of depression. Although we may not find one psychiatrist to agree, we are merely presenting the work of some studies that offer an interesting viewpoint to the disease that one in 20 Americans gets every year. I should say, as well, that anyone who thinks they suffer from depression should, without fail, seek an opinion of someone in the medical field. If you, indeed, suffer from depression or bipolar disorder or schizophrenia, your treatment should not be delayed. I simply encourage you to continually educate yourself on your condition from that point on.

In 1984, W. G. Crook, M. D., published in the *Journal of the American Medical Association* (JAMA) an article called "Depression Associated with Candida Albicans." JAMA is among a handful of the most respected medical journals in the world, but the idea of depression associated with a fungal infection apparently did not catch on.

Listed among the causes of depression you will be challenged to find "diet" or "fungi" as even a remote cause of depression. With the exception of life changes or stress factors, the cause of depression is often linked with genetics, i.e., "it runs in the family." It is difficult, then, to try to answer the question of how a fungus might cause depression. What would a living organism have to do with the way you feel?

You might have read that fungi produce chemicals called myco-toxins. For a refresher, these are chemicals that are released from living fungi for the purpose of killing or harming other organisms that may be competing with the fungus for nutrients. Antibiotics are classic mycotoxins, designed and produced by fungi for killing bacteria. Realizing this, we now manufacture, with the help of fungi, antibiotics in massive quantities each day for the specific purpose of treating bacterial infections. If mycotoxins are designed to do harm, then is it not reasonable to assume that some are more harmful than others? On one hand, for example, penicillin, a very popular mycotoxin, can be consumed by humans. In the proper doses, it is only harmful enough to kill the bacteria that invade our body. On the other hand, if you ever have the misfortune of being exposed to enough *aflatoxin*, you are almost sure to succumb to liver cancer. Some would agree that penicillin is not actually all that harmless; but for sake of example, we'll leave it at that.

If you then take a middle-of-the-road mycotoxin like alcohol, you might expect an immediate effect. Alcohol will kill you, given enough quantity and time, but even in moderation it produces behavioral changes. Once ingested, alcohol is broken down into smaller molecules. One of the chemicals in this degradation pathway is acetaldehyde. If you aren't familiar with this chemical, simply recall yourself or someone you know who has had a hangover. Yes, it is acetaldehyde you have to blame for making you feel so bad. At least now you have someone to blame! So, what are we getting at here?

In an article in the Journal of Nutritional Medicine (1990. 1:33-38), Hunnisett, A., et. al., discuss the "auto-brewery" syndrome. This is a condition whereby carbohydrates ferment in the presence of intestinal microorganisms to yield, you guessed it, alcohol! You don't need to visit a local micro-brewery: you are a walking, talking one yourself! In this study, 69% of the patients who consumed 50 grams of glucose (less than two ounces), about equal to the amount of sugar found in one soft drink, had measurable levels of ethanol (alcohol) in their blood stream only one hour after ingesting the 50 grams of sugar. And what fungus is responsible for the conversion of sugar into alcohol? Right again – brewer's yeast!

If 69 percent of you are fermenting in your intestines every day when you consume potatoes, grains, or beans (carbohydrates), and you are getting alcohol as a by-product in your blood stream, that alcohol has got to break down eventually into the hangover chemical we discussed above. How would you feel if you had to walk around every day in a constant hangover? Do you feel as though you *are* walking around every day in a constant hangover? If you are, you feel pretty depressed.

Do you see where the chronic fatigue syndrome comes into play as well as depression? If you were an alcoholic, you can deduce that it would be best to avoid not only the alcohol but also the excess sugars and carbohydrates in your diet, lest you continue to feed your body the fuel it needs to produce the alcohol.

What if alcohol were not your problem, "auto-brewery" or not? What if you were ingesting one of these toxins directly from the food you were eating? Not unheard of: Schumacher, et. al. (Vet. Hum. Toxicology, February 1995. 37 [1]:39-45), looked at the role of the fumonism B1 toxin, produced by the mold *Fusarium moniliforme*, in causing duodenitis/proximal jejunitis syndrome (DPJ). DPJ is a disease characterized by depression and severe gastric reflux. Do you suffer from both depression and heartburn? Well, the cause of DPJ, a disease of horses, is unknown, but when horses in this study were fed grain contaminated with this fungus, they were able to find evidence of intestinal and liver damage in the horses.

Other mycotoxins, such as T2, vomitoxin, and aflatoxin, found in grain feed containing mold, are well known to cause either weight loss or decreased appetite. Weight loss and changes in appetite are typical symptoms associated with depression. Could exposure to these fungi, or others, be a factor in your symptoms? We will never know unless we begin to test for these chemicals in your blood stream. Please let me know if you find a laboratory in the United States willing to accurately run fungal tests!

There are means by which fungi can directly invade the meninges, or the lining of the brain and spinal cord. Meningitis is nearly always associated with behavioral changes. Most resources will tell you that such an infection, like candidal meningitis, is a devastating and rapidly fatal condition, but other fungi like Histoplasma can have a course of infection than spans a period of years (C. C. Kibbler. 1996).

If you recall the chapter on bowel diseases, you will remember that many people with conditions like irritable bowel syndrome or Crohn's disease have neurologic manifestations as well. Most commonly, they suffer from depression! Could invasion from intestinal yeast into the blood stream or production of mycotoxins by these abundant yeast be the reason for depression? Don't let anyone tell you that yeast cannot invade the blood stream from the bowels. A. G. Prentice (Mycoses. 32 [Suppl. 2]. 42-46. 1989) stated that "even without any other predisposing factor, overgrowth of Candida in the gut will lead to invasion of the blood stream."

Studies and evidence aside, most people who seek help from someone like Doug present with some degree of loss of energy and many have been previously diagnosed with depression. As far as I am aware, nearly one-hundred percent (100%) of these people respond favorably to changes in their diet and elimination of yeast and yeast-contaminated products in their diet. And to me, if it quacks like a duck and walks like a duck, it is a duck! You don't call a cure of depression with diet changes and elimination of yeast a coincidence; you call it a treatment. And you call the cause of depression not genetics, but either a poor diet or a fungus.

Bygone Days:
A Depression Treatment that Worked

by Doug A. Kaufmann

In the late 1970s, I opened one of the very first laboratories in the United States that dealt with the disease process as though it were nutritionally based. By the second year of operations, our gross income exceeded $1,000,000. During this time, I worked around the clock. I ran tests, made sales calls, did my own books, and cleaned the toilets. Rarely was I home. To say I was stressed was a gross understatement.

A friend suggested that I take a supplement called L-tryptophan to relieve my stress. I began taking this small pill twice daily and the change was noticeable and incredible. No, my job did not lighten up, but it seemed as though my body was fully relaxed and life was more enjoyable. My brain began to work in unison with my body! Knowing that such a feeling could be addictive, I used the L-tryptophan on an "as needed" basis only, and it never let me down. I recommended it to thousands of people.

L-tryptophan works by causing a natural elevation of the neurotransmitter seratonin in the pineal gland of the brain. When this neurochemical is elevated, peace and calm are promoted. Thousands of medical documents have confirmed that, indeed, this simple amino acid found in milk, egg whites, and turkey assists the body in producing calmness. Many doctors and nutritionists began putting their patients on L-tryptophan, and several of my psychiatrist friends used it to treat depression in their patients. Most commonly, L-tryptophan was used to induce peaceful sleep and dreams. It was simply a wonder supplement. And then something horrible happened.

A foreign supplier of this harmless amino acid supplement shipped a tainted batch to the U. S. Some individuals got very sick while taking the supplement. Others died of a condition called eosinophilia-myalgia syndrome (EMS). All of the people who suffered and died were taking L-tryptophan supplied from the tainted batch from this one Japanese firm. The Food and Drug Administration (FDA) immediately ordered all L-tryptophan supplements, no matter who manufactured them, off the market. There were several safe suppliers. This move seemed harsh since more people continue to die each year from over-the-counter aspirin than ever died from the tainted tryptophan.

In a startling move, the FDA allowed pharmacies to continue carrying L-tryptophan, but no longer could American citizens get this natural supplement over the counter. The bottle I used to pay $7 for now became available only following a doctor's office visit and a $40 prescription – a $100 investment. Finding a physician sympathetic to their patient's self-medicating needs became almost impossible. Worse, physicians were warned of the extreme dangers of having their patients use this amino acid that had maimed and killed.

At exactly the same time, the FDA was finalizing their approval of a new drug that artifically elevated the pineal gland neurochemical seratonin. It seems as though this seratonin runs through naturally occurring cycles throughout the day. It is produced in higher quantities when you are resting and sleeping and lower quantities when active. What this new FDA-approved drug, Prozac, did was readjust this natural cycle and inhibited the "reuptake" of seratonin whenever the pill was taken. What neither this drug, nor any other pharmaceutical drug on the market, has been able to do is to stimulate seratonin naturally and safely.

One might guess, therefore, that L-tryptophan, available from health food stores without prescription, was a hindrance to the makers of a group of pharmaceutical drugs called selective seratonin reuptake inhibitors (SSRI). Man could not replicate what God had provided naturally. There are now numerous SSRIs produced by several drug manufacturers. With the safe and natural L-tryptophan off the shelves of health food stores, a billion-dollar pharmaceutical bonanza was created. Prozac was FDA approved only four days after L-tryptophan was taken out of health food stores.

That was some 13 years ago. Today, many physicians don't even remember the scare that was created. It is likely that if you educate your doctor on the safety of this amino acid, he or she may write a prescription for you. Remember that L-tryptophan has a nutrient co-factor and should always be taken with 25 to 50 mg of vitamin B6.

Whereas your doctor may have forgotten the scare, your pharmacist may be another story. Pharmacists have wonderful memories, and most will not even carry this simple amino acid for fear of hurting you. Imagine that!!! Call around and find a compounding pharmacist in your area. They will provide you with L-tryptophan.

L-tryptophan was a wonderful breakthrough for depression sufferers. It seemed very unusual to me that the FDA would pull something off of the entire market because one foreign batch was tainted. It seemed even more unusual to me that 96 hours later a billion dollar pharmaceutical industry was created based on the success of this remarkable natural amino acid.

Food, Fungus, and the Forlorn Patient

by Milt Gearing, Ph.D.

Almost any mental health professional will openly admit that the physiological causes of depression are not well understood. We do not know exactly what enables many antidepressant medications to work for specific patients, although we do know that they are effective in treating depression. Why does any given antidepressant work for some depressed patients and not for others? Why do some antidepressants work for a while on many depressed patients and then quit working? There are plausible theories offered as answers to many of these questions, but none of these theories has been proven.

During my years as a clinical psychologist, I have seen many patients who present with severe depression. Some of these patients have responded extremely well to antidepressant medication, while other patients have not. Since I have started working with Doug Kaufmann, both for my family's health and the health of my patients, I have referred to him some of my patients who suffer from depression.

All of these patients had tried antidepressant medications and gained little or no relief from them. All had worked in psychotherapy and made progress, yet each continued to be weighed down with serious symptoms of depression.

These patients were taken off all antidepressant medications and placed on the Initial Phase Diet (IPD), a low carbohydrate antifungal diet and program. All of these people have since shown amazing improvement in their depressive symptoms and a welcomed return to a normal lifestyle.

How is this possible? Some research in recent years has actually discovered a link between depression and diet. One of the best articles on this subject is called "Carbohydrates and Depression" (Wurtman, Richard J. and Wurtman, Judith J. *Scientific American*. January 1989. Pp. 68-75). One of the diet-related links to depression discussed by this article involves the tendency of sufferers from "carbohydrate-craving obesity" to consume excessive amounts of carbohydrates in order to improve their mood!

Just the opposite is true according to other authors. The landmark article by W. G. Crook, M.D., called "Depression Associated with Candida Albicans" (discussed by David A. Holland, M.D., in his article in this chapter) described a direct link between food consumed (carbohydrates) and depression symptoms in Candida (yeast) patients.

While there are many causes and many effective treatments for depression, those patients who do not respond to conventional treatments and who do show Candida symptoms should consider the benefits that the Candida diet and antifungal program could offer them for their depression. This approach has worked wonders!

Pain, Depression, and Fungus

A Testimonial
by H. H., Dallas, Texas

One would probably say that I am a happy, confident individual. I have not always been, however, the confident person that I am today. My life has been a roller coaster of ups and downs. As a teenager, I suffered from depression and eating disorders. At 13, dealing with both ailments, I tried to commit suicide. In the later years of my teens and into my 20s, my mood swings and low self esteem cost me many jobs. Never did I link the two with the foods that I ate. As a matter of fact, I realized the relation to depression and irritability only two days ago!

I began seeing Doug Kaufmann to relieve painful tendonitis symptoms. After two weeks of following Doug's Initial Phase Diet, the tendonitis greatly improved. With the help of holiday baking I "fell off the wagon" for about 16 hours. Once I had my first bite of sugar, I began my binge. I ate, and ate, and ate. Several things happened. I craved more food, my arm started hurting again, and my sinus problems came back again. Most importantly, that old depressed and irritable feeling that I have struggled with for so long came back.

That night and the following day I was extremely moody. Any little thing filled me with anger. I felt impatient, anxious, mad

93

at my lack of control, and mad at my husband because he didn't do things the way "I" wanted them done. He and I had a little "tiff" because of my anger and sarcasm.

Looking back over this "challenge" day of eating sugars has helped my husband and me see the true meaning of the statement, "You are what you eat." He and I went back on the Initial Phase Diet immediately, and within just a few hours I could feel a difference. I can now focus my thoughts and my mood swings are gone.

Chapter Six

Relating Fungus to Dermatology

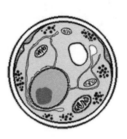

Skin Disorders and Fungus

by Doug A. Kaufmann

Dr. David R. Weakley was a Johns Hopkin's medical school graduate and professor of dermatology at Southwestern Medical School. In 1988, Dr. Weakley and I began working together at Medical City Dallas – a very large medical building, hospital, and medical theme park all rolled into one. Within a short time, Dr. Weakley had two other dermatologists working in his office. All was well as I set out to learn more about dermatology and they set out to add nutrition into their rather large dermatology practice. We would work closely together for five years.

Dr. Weakley was astonished with the many symptoms over and above general dermatology that we were able to reverse when using a dietary approach to skin conditions. I recall him being concerned that dermatologists were able to fix migraine headaches, bowel problems, and depression. Had he crossed a line in medicine? How could a skin doctor fix arthritis – a joint problem? I remember telling him that first and foremost he was a physician who took an oath to help people. Second, it was his medical establishment that had decided to compartmentalize the human body. He should be proud of his new abilities to get people better, no matter what they suffered from!

But along with this new pride came politicking. I remember insurance companies withholding payments to him because he tested his skin patients for food allergy. Their concern must have seemed logical to insurance companies. Why not rub some cortisone on it and charge $35? I would argue that 100 visits at $35 each for prescribing cortisone actually costs $3,500 – and the problem hasn't been fixed! Yet, we were able to transcend routine dermatology in reversing not only skin problems, but also numerous other problems for which these patients saw many doctors!

Soon, Dr. Weakley began fighting back. He wrote many letters demanding payments for services that he had rendered. He then apprised the insurance giants that dictated his practice (this is quite common today) that the monies that they had been dumping in gastroenterologists, gynecologists, internists, and rheumatologists offices could come to a screeching halt. He had been able to fix all of those problems by incorporating nutrition into his practice. You would think they would be thrilled! Yet the financial harassment not only persisted, but actually accelerated.

Prior to his death in 1995, Dr. Weakley and I learned a great deal about the role of food allergies in dermatological conditions. We used a blood test to detect food allergies. Although today this is commonly done, in 1988 we were pioneers. Some years earlier I had discovered the root cause of most food allergy, and Dr. Weakley was impressed with these findings. During our first few years together, we tested patients for food allergy in order to confirm that they did, indeed, exist in dermatology patients. If so, Dr. Weakley would often write a prescription for antifungal medicines to test my theory. And why antifungal prescriptions for food allergy? You will find this interesting!

One of my mentors in medical science was Dr. Everett Hughes, with whom I worked on a limited basis at USC Medical School. We had collaborated on several research papers that Dr. Hughes had published in the scientific literature. I did the food allergy tests and he interpreted this data, along with other data he gathered, in an effort to confirm that food caused symptoms! One day after a pleasant lunch, Dr. Hughes asked me how food allergy could be so accurately detected in the blood. Did food actually get into the blood? We guessed that undigested foods somehow leaked through the intestine and ended up circulating in the blood. Although this sounded terribly illogical, it was the best that we had in the 1970s.

Some years later, I read a research paper entitled, "Antigenically intact food macromolecules exiting the gut lumen." This paper confirmed my suspicions that small pieces of undigested foods, still intact, leaked through tiny holes in the intestinal wall and gained access to the blood stream. Once there, a type of white blood cell (B-cell lymphocyte) recognizes the food particle as foreign, forms an antibody protein against the food, thus rendering it harmless from causing damage inside the body. After the food particle combines with the B-cell antibody protein, these tiny "micro-food-chips" are referred to as either "antigen antibody complexes" or "immune complexes." These complexes are then filtered out of the body.

Throughout the years, I stopped worrying about food allergy. Yes, it does exist and yes, I am one of the individuals credited with starting the "food allergy revolution" in the 1970s. But testing for food allergies is, in my opinion, not really necessary anymore. I am less concerned about food leaking through the intestines than I am with my concern as to why holes exist in the intestinal wall. And what about the normal inhabitants of the intestines leaking out? Remember that there are yeasts and bacteria inside the intestines and should these be allowed to cross the intestinal barrier, problems significantly worse than food allergy would soon surface.

Septicemia is the word used to describe blood poisoning by bacteria. *Fungemia* applies to fungus gaining access to the blood. In either case, doctors will sound the alarm when these conditions are known or even thought to exist. Now I am certainly not a doctor, but I have always wondered how bacterial infections spread, if not via the blood stream. And I have often pondered why antibiotic and antifungal medicines are **systemic medicines** (actions occur by the medicines crossing the gut-blood barrier and the blood-organ barrier) given the general medical consensus that these microorganisms would kill a person if they ever got into the blood. Yet I constantly hear, "My doctor said that fungus could never get into my blood stream because it would have killed me if it had." I dare say it is confusing!

You will find that *septicemia* and *fungemia* are most likely quite common, unbeknownst to most physicians. In 1963, Harold Hyman, M.D., the prominent author of a medical encyclopedia, stated that approximately one-half of the population of the United States had suffered from a systemic fungal disorder that had largely gone unnoticed[1]. How could this be if fungus would kill a person if it ever gained access to their blood stream? Has the population of the U.S. decreased by 50% since 1963, or have medical doctors learned wrong information in most medical schools? Hmmm.

Finally, while we're on the subject of skin, just how many skin conditions do food and fungus cause? I believe *all* of them, but you'll be hard pressed to find one dermatologist who credits *any* skin symptom or disease to food or fungus. Do skin patients really suffer from steroid medication deficiency after all? I would challenge any physician and certainly any specializing in dermatology, to take the Kaufmann challenge. Yes, I believe that acne, rosacea, psoriasis, dandruff, hives, and eczema, to name a few, intimately link food with fungus. No, the dermatological organizations do not concur.

1. Hyman, Harold. The Complete Home Medical Encyclopedia. 1963.

The Science of Skin Fungus

by David A. Holland, M.D.

As you already know if you've been listening to Doug, the skin is the largest organ in the body. It serves many functions, the least of which is to protect you from outside invaders. Most importantly, it keeps our insides from becoming outsides! Everything is neatly tucked into our body by nature of the skin. What you may also know, then, if you are a faithful Doug Kaufmann "roadie," is that the skin may serve as a signal of deeper processes occurring inside of your body. In fact, skin lesions are at times the earliest clue to the fact that one has a systemic mycoses, or internal fungal infection (C. C. Kibbler, 1996). What we've found out is that fungus may cause problems with both the insides and the outsides.

Part of the claim to fame of fungi is that they were actually the first microorganisms shown to cause an infection or disease in humans. Specifically, it was a fungus called *Trichophyton schoenleinii* (you'll be quizzed on this later!) that caused skin infections in humans (*Principles and Practice of Clinical Mycology*. Kibbler, C. C., John Wiley and Sons, Ltd. 1996.). This being the case, you'd think that everyone would know about the ubiquity of fungi. Not so, however. Southwestern Medical Center, one of the most prestigious medical centers (in our area, at least), touts the fact that they receive $150,000,000 annually in research grants, yet they do not staff *one* mycologist

among their hundreds of scientists and physicians. It is a
similar story across the country: not many mycologists actually
exist. It is no wonder that the role of fungi is often overlooked
and that the extent that fungi play in skin disease is commonly
unknown.

One of the more familiar groups of fungi is the dermatophytes.
These usually cause only superficial infections, such as "jock
itch" or toenail fungus. A dermatophyte infection of the skin is
also known as "ringworm." Fungal infections of the skin are
one of the most common infectious diseases in the world with
an estimated 10% to 15% of the entire world's population
being infected with these (C. C. Kibbler)! The sources of these
fungi are many: soil, animals, human contact, and plants.

Sometimes these supposedly superficial infections can cause
symptoms in parts of the body distal to the part that is actually
infected. For example, one may have a terrible athlete's foot or
toenail infection and then suddenly break out in a rash on the
palm of the hand. We call these "id reactions." The rash on the
hand is not due to the athlete's foot, but rather from the mycotoxins (fungal poisons) released by the athlete's foot fungus
into one's bloodstream. These, in turn, affect the palms of the
hands. The palm rash is due to the toxins, not the foot fungus,
per se.

There are other ways that skin fungi are able to affect the body
internally. Through a non-official poll, we found that many
patients with toenail fungus coincidentally also had elevated
blood cholesterol levels. Then, once the toenail fungus was

treated with an antifungal, the cholesterol reduced! (British Medical Journal. 1995. 311:919-22). By deduction, this would mean without a doubt that the fungus contributed to the high cholesterol. Costantini (1994) has found research explaining how fungal toxins (mycotoxins) exposed to the blood stream caused an elevation in that person's blood cholesterol as a protective measure: cholesterol binds fungal toxins, thereby rendering them less harmful. Get rid of the fungus, then, and your body won't need the excess cholesterol.

On the flip side, we have seen how internal fungal infections contribute externally to skin diseases and symptoms. Persons with coccidiomycoses or blastomycosis (infections of the lungs) may suffer from a variety of skin lesions. Some may even resemble skin cancer (C. C. Kibbler)! Candida albicans, a yeast that is found in nearly every single normal, healthy person, can not only cause external skin infections, like diaper rash and perleche (manifested as dry, red, cracked skin at the corners of the mouth), but it may also contribute to internal problems like vaginal yeast infections and intestinal problems.

There are still other skin diseases, like psoriasis, acne, hives, and eczema, which don't seem to have such an obvious relation to any internal infection. However, people have been treated empirically (treatment based on experience vs. evidence) for internal yeast or fungal infections and have the external problems go away as well. There is a collection of literature showing that psoriasis is indeed a fungal infection, caused by either the fungus itself or, as we discussed above, caused by the fungal toxins released into the blood stream (Costantini, 1994).

This literature has been supported by many personal testimonials of people who were treated for fungal infections and were "cured" of their psoriasis. (I used the quotes because psoriasis is supposedly incurable, but I beg to differ!)

The internal problem in most cases is preventable. Usually it is caused by a diet high in refined carbohydrates and yeast foods and/or exposure to certain drugs, like antibiotics, steroids, or birth control pills. For example, there hasn't been a child that suffers from eczema that I have met who hasn't been exposed to antibiotics in one way or another at an early age. At other times, the internal problem has been a result of inhaling fungal spores and succumbing to a systemic fungal infection, regardless of how healthy you were to begin with. Remember, an external fungal infection can always be a sign that something more serious and devastating is happening inside of your body. To that end, even things like toenail fungus should not be taken lightly.

If you happen to be one who suffers from a chronic skin ailment, especially if no one has been able to offer relief or cure, the possibility exists that you would respond to a combination of a change in diet and either natural or pharmaceutical antifungal remedies. As always, "you are what you eat." So, your diet is going to play the most profound role in long term relief.

The Kaufmann Challenge

by Doug A. Kaufmann

Now that we've whetted your appetite and piqued your interest, let me make a broad generalization about the medical field. In my 25 years of studying nutrition, I have never seen any one specialty in medicine that loves big words like I have seen in dermatology. To be perfectly frank with you, I can't pronounce them all, but I'll just bet that a good dermatologist can! The problem remains that there is a vast difference in the ability to pronounce big words and to cure big problems. Would you rather your dermatologist pronounce them or reverse them?

In his excellent dissertation on skin fungus problems, Dr. Holland mentioned that empirical evidence (the body's response to a treatment) sometimes proves stronger than logic. Again, please understand that the information here should never replace an initial physical visit with a dermatologist when you have skin problems. If that doctor gives you the clean bill of health or recommends a treatment that you are not comfortable with, please tell him! Just call the nurse and leave a message that you're going to try something for 30 days and if this something doesn't work, you'll be back to visit again. Many of you will have positive results with this program, and that may well be the way to educate doctors! Imagine if three or four of their patients called them back and said, "This is something you need to learn!"

Here's how I'd begin investigating the role of food and fungus in my skin condition, if I were an otherwise healthy adult:

1. Unless otherwise directed by a physician, eat only meat, poultry, fish, vegetables (no potatoes, corn, or beans),
   ✳ green apples, grapefruit, berries, eggs (never break the yolk while cooking these), nuts (except peanuts), and
   — seeds. Eat no sugars, bread, grains, or pasta.
2. Drink eight to ten ounces of fresh-squeezed organic
   ✳ carrot juice twice daily and in this "cocktail" place one teaspoon of apple cider vinegar.
3. Take two caprylic acid tablets three times a day.
4. Stop taking all unnecessary supplements and retain only those that were absolutely necessary.

If acne were my problem, I would call 1-800-914-8888 and order the "Healthwise" facial dip kit and use as directed.

If I had bowel symptoms, especially constipation, I'd take one heaping tablespoon of psyllium hulls in a small jar of water (4 — to 5 oz.), shake well, and drink quickly. I'd do this each night just before bed.

— —This program may worsen the skin problem for the first few days, but continuation should cause remission within a short time. You might try this program for 30 days. Take a Polaroid picture of yourself prior to initiation and then again in 30 days. If you see a vast difference (and are fully dressed), share these pictures with your friends and doctors. You deserve to have great skin, and they deserve this information.

Chapter Seven

Relating Fungus to Heart Health

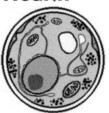

The Heart of the Matter ... Is It Fungus?

by Doug A. Kaufmann

Do you recall what you did yesterday? Fifteen hundred individuals cannot recall what happened in their lives yesterday – because they lost their lives to a heart attack. Thousands more are crippled each day from cardiac complications. Heart disease is the major cause of death in this advanced medical arena we call the United States.

There are no shortages of "experts" and published medical research papers confirming that cardiac disease is a killer. But if they are all right, why do the deaths and statistics just keep climbing? Are we not heeding their expert advice, or are the experts wrong?

Pick up any nutritional book, speak with any cardiologist, or call the American Heart Association – each will confirm that cigarette smoking, high cholesterol, and diet cause heart disease. You will not, however, find what I believe to be the true cause of heart disease from any of the "experts." Sometimes "experts," even in alternative health care, are blind when it comes to the cause of heart disease. A respected alternative medical book expounding solely upon heart disease was published in 1997 and features many prominent alternative physicians. Again, we see nothing more than a compilation of nutritional articles and nutritional therapies. There is not a word on fungus or yeast in this entire book. If you don't understand what causes something, your conclusions on how to reverse it are moot. Sometimes you stumble onto a treatment that actually works. You might now be wondering if natural cardiac strengtheners like CoQ_{10}, grape seed extracts, and hawthorne berries are actually antifungals. I'm proud of you!

I believe that a sedentary lifestyle causes heart disease. Our bodies were meant to move! I agree that diet contributes to heart disease, but I disagree as to which foods in the diet are contributors. I believe that wheat, corn, potatoes, and sugar have far more to do with coronary disease than bacon and eggs. Although it is virtually impossible to find any one referring to this, I believe that alcoholic beverages cause more heart disease than pure, unadulterated dairy products (try to find those!). In essence, I believe that low fat diets being promoted by dieticians and heart associations are responsible for keeping them in business! Low fat means high sugar!

And cigarette smoking? In 1968, a researcher by the name of Bock discovered that fresh cut tobacco leaves did **not** induce cancer, but cured tobacco (a proprietary process used by the tobacco companies that purportedly adds yeast and sugars to the tobacco) **did** induce cancer. So it appears that the tobacco industry may be making their product hazardous to our health – even without their knowledge. And what industry could possibly win by having cigarettes so full of dangerous fermented yeast and sugar?!

Now you ask, "OK, Doug. What does cancer have to do with heart disease?" It is my opinion that the same thing that causes cancer also causes heart disease – and many other diseases in man. Since I figured this out many years ago, there has been nothing more frustrating than observing the actions of the American Heart Association (AHA), a fund raising organization that raises money by selling its name to food producers. Pick up a box of many of today's popular multi-colored or frosted cereals and you will notice a stamp of approval from the AHA. Do you sincerely believe that the AHA is acting in the public's best interest by "endorsing" these sugar laden products? It is time for Americans to stand up and realize that when money is involved there are smaller moral standards and larger bank deposits.

The powerful AHA is not alone. Presently, the American Cancer Society (ACS) and even the American Medical Association (AMA) sell their names – in the public's "best interest," of course! [Editor's Note: Fortunately, the AMA recently rescinded their contract with Sunbeam, a manufacturer of medical products.] We're on our own, kids. And we'd better learn how to take care of our heart health, because there is no shortage of for-profit hospitals that gleefully endorse these glorified fund raising activities.

If you suffer from any number of heart conditions, it is imperative to be evaluated by a physician first and foremost. Most likely, medicines and/or surgery will be prescribed. As it is in all areas of medicine, not just cardiology, it is unfortunate that many doctors have no concept of how invasive the fungal infections really are.

The Heart of Fungus

by David Holland, M.D.

It seems these days that there are only two things to die of: a heart attack or terminal cancer. Granted, there are many more sad ways one can leave this cruel world, but on our healthy quest we probably think of these two ways as our prime enemies. I mean, these are what we want to prevent while on our mission to a healthy life, aren't they – along with a disease-free life and a quality existence? Preventing these diseases is something that is in my hands – my control, to the extent that God allows. And even then, who knows when I'll be struck down by a truck (I do live in Texas, remember). But while I'm here, I'd like to take my best shot at living a healthy life, wouldn't you?

Now, when we speak of heart problems, what do we think of most often? That big word "cholesterol," right? Haven't we been pounded into thinking that cholesterol has something to do with either preventing or succumbing to a heart attack? The trendy word for cholesterol is "fat." Low fat this and low fat that – I'm so sick of "low fat" that I'm beginning to experience chest pains. Years ago doctors recognized the fact that some people with heart problems, specifically atherosclerosis ("hardening of the arteries," from now on referred to as <u>coronary artery disease</u>, or <u>CAD</u>), had extremely elevated serum cholesterol levels. From then on, cholesterol became an immediate enemy. What is worse is that they assumed that if our serum cholesterol was high, we must have been getting extraordinary amounts in our diets – we were "pigging out!"

So, out the cholesterol came – excommunicated from good food as we know it. The question now is, "Does cholesterol, a natural substance found in every human cell, directly contribute to plaque in my arteries?" Did you know in over half of the subjects suffering from heart attacks, the victims had normal cholesterol levels? Enough of this: let me put down my fat free Hershey's Chocolate Syrup and let's tackle this subject.

I first direct you to the work of Professor A. V. Costantini, M.D., retired head, World Health Organization Collaborating Center for Mycotoxins in Foods, who took 18 years of his life, at his own expense, to dig up every article he could find on fungi, mycotoxins, and their relation to CAD. He put his collection together into a book (Fungalbionics: Atherosclerosis. 1994. ISBN #3-930939-00-2). Good luck trying to get this book here in the U.S. of A. It wouldn't be a very popular book with certain establishments here. In his conclusion of this collection, Dr. Costantini states, "There is a known cause of atherosclerosis and that cause is the fungi and their mycotoxins." He also summarizes that there is, indeed, a food relation to the cause of CAD, but it is only food that has been contaminated with fungi and/or the mycotoxins they produce. The information presented in this book is overwhelming, and way beyond the scope of our discussion now; but suffice it to say it puts the question of what causes atherosclerosis to rest.

One study (*New England Journal of Medicine.* 03 April 1997.) looked at the role of inflammation in the risk of developing atherosclerosis. As is typical, what was not addressed is what caused the inflammation! Always look for the cause not for the sign or symptom. Also, when you look at or hear any new studies that try to address the cause, ask yourself, "Who funded this study?" Remember what I said above: Dr. Costantini researched for 18 years at his own expense, specifically without the funding of pharmaceutical companies. Week after week I hear well-meaning pharmaceutical company representatives present the latest studies on why their drug is better, only to disappointingly find out that their own company funded the study. What do you expect the results to be?! Certainly, they are not going to favor their competition.

What about taking a cholesterol-lowering drug to lower your cholesterol? If you are the less than one percent of people in the U. S. that genetically inherit a tendency to abnormally high cholesterol, I think it may be a good idea. Otherwise, I'd be asking you what are you doing with exercise and diet?

How do these drugs work anyway? A study on one such drug, Lovastatin, showed that it inhibits fungal growth (Antibiot Khimioter. 1996. 41[11]:3-6). On a smaller level, the drug inhibits a certain enzyme involved in the manufacture of cholesterol; but did you know that many cholesterol-lowering drugs were initially studied for the purpose of killing fungi? Perhaps they were more profitable as cholesterol-lowering drugs. Fine with me, as long as they kill those fungi!

Should you even worry about severely high cholesterol? I would! Elevated cholesterol is a response to an invasion by a toxin in your blood stream. Remember Costantini's research (1994) explaining how fungal toxins in the blood stream caused elevated blood cholesterol: cholesterol binds fungal toxins, rendering them less harmful. Rid yourself of the fungus and your body doesn't need the excess cholesterol.

Does your doctor doubt this? Ask him or her what would happen if you took the drug cyclosporine, a drug used to suppress the immune system so your body does not reject an organ transplant. One hundred percent of the time you will develop elevated cholesterol and, subsequently, atherosclerosis -- and also, in some instances, cancer! Cyclosporine, folks, is a mycotoxin – a poison produced by a fungus and used as a drug.

Several mycotoxins are found in foods such as corn, peanuts, beer, barley, hay, apples, and wheat. The steak you are not eating is less likely to be bad because of the meat and fat than it is because the cattle ate moldy feed, complete with fungal poisons. Those poisons are now stored in the fat! I'm not sure how to get around this to eat the meat safely, but fiber in vegetables do bind mycotoxins; so be sure to eat fresh veggies or use a psyllium fiber supplement when you eat that meat. [Editor's note: range-fed beef have almost **no** mycotoxins or dangerous E. coli bacteria.]

"Don't they screen for toxins in grains?" you might ask. They sure do, and we know of one such laboratory. But we do not have a zero tolerance for mycotoxins in grains in the U.S. It would be cost prohibitive. We only routinely screen for seven of the several hundred known mycotoxins. You would nearly have to quit eating to completely avoid every source of mold and mycotoxin. But you can be wary of the more "notorious" foods like corn, peanuts, and beer. I will give you one hint on beer: they tend to use the poorer quality, often moldy, grains for producing beer. (Counsel for Agricultural Science and Technology. Report 116. Nov 1989.) Just think about that as you wonder why alcohol is implicated in so many diseases! And please, folks, unless you have one of those rare disorders with cholesterol, eat those raw nuts (all but peanuts) and eggs (cooked with yolk unbroken), like Doug keeps telling you.

A 1960 American Cancer Society study showed those who consumed **more** than five eggs per week had *fewer* heart attacks and stroke deaths than those who ate **less** than five eggs per week ("Eggs are Great Food." Joseph Hattersley. *Townsend Letter for Doctors and Patients.* January, 1996). Try to eat eggs cooked with the yolks intact (Gary Price Todd, M.D.). Another study in the mid-1970s concluded that you could cut your risk of heart attack by 50%, 60% if you are a woman, by eating nuts five or more times per week. Naturally, we're not talking about the honey-roasted variety nor those roasted in peanut oil!

Let me give you my take on this: I am pretty convinced that oxidation in the blood stream or cholesterol in and of itself has little to do with atherosclerosis. The plaque which is responsible for causing blockage of the arteries and subsequent heart attacks is a complex formation of a cell known as "granuloma."

Never mind the long word, but the formation of a granuloma in the body requires the presence of a foreign substance – either a "bug," like a fungus, or a metal or toxin, like a mycotoxin. Cholesterol is not a foreign substance. Neither is oxidation a foreign process, but rather one that is used by our body to perform normal, daily protective functions. And I do think that if you are a fervent exerciser it is OK to eat up the carbohydrates; but if you are either sick or are among the ranks of couch potatoes, I think that the ever-popular low fat, high carbohydrate diet is one of the most harmful things for your body.

Excess carbohydrates, which are, in more simple terms, sugars, are stored as fat inside your body. Declaring across the board that every one should eat low fat is to say that we are all equal. Look at the size and shape of different people. Do you really think one diet is right for every one of us? Of course you don't. That is exactly why there will always be a battle as to which diet is better. If you are unwell, though, I'd lose the carbs!

~~~~~

CASE PRESENTATIONS

These are three cases that Doug and I, personally, worked with. Take note of these numbers!

Case No. 1

A 37 year old male with a triglyceride (serum fatty acid) level of 342 (normal is less than 200) and a total cholesterol level of 237 (normal is less than 200). HDL, or good cholesterol, was low at 30, and LDL, or bad cholesterol, was high at 139. His doctor advised a low fat diet, weight reduction, and a recheck of the blood tests in two months.

After two months on a low fat diet, his triglycerides shot up to 703 and total cholesterol reduced slightly to 224, but his HDL fell even lower, to 25, losing its protective effect, and his LDL was not measurable because his triglycerides were so high. At this point we saw him, advised a high protein diet with high-unsaturated fats (i.e., raw nuts and avocados) and low carbohydrates. His blood fats normalized within two weeks.

Case No. 2

A 30-something year old male with triglycerides exceeding 1,000 and cholesterol over 300. Within ten days of starting a low carbohydrate diet, his triglycerides plummeted to 160 (normal) and his cholesterol dropped to 205. He was one happy camper!

Case No. 3

A 50+ year old male with cholesterol of 293, triglycerides of 350. Two weeks after starting the program mentioned above, he had a cholesterol of 198 (normal) and triglycerides of 226 – well on its way to being normal.

Why I Can No Longer Sleep In On Saturday Mornings!

by Nathan L. Lipton, M.D.

After working all week as a busy opthalmologist, I look forward to being able to sleep in on Saturday mornings. Well, Doug Kaufmann put an end to that! Several months ago, while lying in bed one Saturday morning, enjoying the freedom of not having to get up, I happened to begin listening to the radio. I tuned in to 94.9 "The Word," a station I often enjoy for its spiritual content. That's when I first heard the excited, enthusiastic voice of Doug Kaufmann blasting the medical profession for over-treating everyone with antibiotics and other assorted sins that we physicians commit. I quickly found myself listening intently and even agreeing with much of what I heard.

I am a board-certified opthalmologist in practice for 20 years. I treat patients of all ages and specialize in laser vision correction and surgery for cross-eyed children. But I certainly know that we doctors don't have all the answers. Because I am intently interested in alternative medicine, I have always been open to learning about all facets of health from whatever sources I could find. I had listened to other health and nutrition-oriented shows, but "Your Health Matters" was different! I knew I was hooked when, the following Saturday, I set my clock for 7:00 a.m. to catch Doug's program from the beginning to the end.

Although I feel that Western medicine as practiced in this
country is the most advanced in the world, I have recognized
for many years the importance of nutrition as the foundation for
health. My two favorite quotes on this subject are:

*The doctor of the future will give no medicine,
but will interest his patient in the care of the human frame,
in diet, and in the cause and prevention of disease.*
— Thomas Edison

~~~~~

Our food should be our medicine.
Our medicine should be our food.
— Hippocrates

Besides being one of millions of Doug Kaufmann radio listen-
ers, I have also gotten to know Doug as a friend. Not surprisingly, he is just as terrific off the air. What really comes across
with Doug is his sincerity and how much he cares about
helping people. For me, Doug also fulfills the role of teacher; I
am constantly learning from him. I am honored to have been
asked to contribute to this section.

Heart Disease and Diet

by Doug A. Kaufmann

Atherosclerosis means "clogging of the arteries." Like most diseases in America, the cause is unknown but the treatments are many. This chapter is dedicated to every individual who has ever thought they were having a heart attack and really weren't. Had you known that the meal you just finished was actually the cause of those horrible symptoms, you could have relaxed a little. Instead, you went to the doctor, had a physical exam, and were informed that your heart was just fine.

Which diet is the best one to prevent the symptoms that mimic heart attack? Heart disease is often a symptom of a complex event taking place within your body. Parasitic fungus can gain access to your heart and circulatory system and cause irregular events within the body. Since the fungus is parasitic, it requires certain foods to feed it. Fungus craves carbohydrates like potatoes, pasta, and bread. So, the next time you pull your car off the road and worry about that impending heart attack, take a moment and review what you just ate. It is likely that this review will have you knowing that your diet must change!

Chapter Eight

Relating Fungus to Allergies

The Fungal Link to Allergies

by Doug A. Kaufmann

The year was 1972. I had just been honorably discharged from
the U. S. Navy after serving a turbulent, albeit rewarding, four
years. I was now trained in acute care medicine. I was disillu-
sioned because those four years had likely resulted in the loss
of a formal medical education. I really did want to become a
physician, but had neither the grade point average nor my youth
to support me through medical school. I resumed my college
studies in Los Angeles and began working with an ear, nose,
and throat allergist. Dr. Howard Gottschalk was one of the
finest men I have ever met in the course of my medical career.

Like health maintenance organizations today, the military
herded patients through like cattle. At my tender age, I truly
believed that this was as good as it got in health care. Dr.
Gottschalk would provide the integrity catalyst that I so desper-
ately needed to witness in medicine. He absolutely loved his
patients and, of equal importance, they absolutely loved him.

I became certified by the American Society of Allergy Techni-
cians (ASAT) in 1973 and worked with Dr. Gottschalk for six
years in that capacity. He was a visionary who instinctively
knew the future of medicine. Within two years of my employ-
ment, he sent me to the Washington University School of
Medicine in St. Louis to research food allergy. Food allergy,

mind you, was extremely controversial. Within a year of returning home from St. Louis, the allergists across the street from our small office would "educate" the public that food allergy was extremely rare, affecting perhaps only a miniscule percentage of the population. I am certain that we represented competition to them, and they wanted to squelch this concept of food allergy as quickly as possible.

You see, the concept of food allergy involves a resolution of two medical hurdles. If immune reactions to food *did* cause disease, the general public might be able to bypass a doctor's visit and recover by changing their diet. Simply changing dietary patterns would seemingly "cure" the affliction, if food allergy existed. This was unspeakable in 1975. No one could possibly self-diagnose! Additionally, doctors are not taught nutrition in medical school. If food really did cause symptoms and diseases, an admission would have to be made that something was sorely lacking in medical schools. I believe the term my sons use to dispel this notion would be "fat chance." As we all know, doctors learn *everything* in medical school!

The erroneous information that the allergists were dispensing never daunted Dr. Gottschalk, who was immune to perpetuating medicine solely for turf protection. For me, however, this was a new concept. Those of you who have followed my work through the years know that today I am undaunted by medical deception, just as Dr. Gottschalk was in 1975. Today, it seems, misleading the general public has become the standard. The miniature print on pharmaceutical drug advertisements, in my opinion, represents only one form of lying or deception.

Allergy is defined as an adverse reaction to an otherwise harmless agent. Foods, animal danders, pollens, dusts, and molds are otherwise harmless agents. Many allergists today still contend that food allergy is quite rare, yet most will skin test their patients for foods. I've often wondered why this is done when their own academy denies that food allergy exists in all but a small portion of the entire population. Certainly, allergists are not just in it for the money! Most of them must really believe that food allergy is a problem or they just wouldn't skin test for foods.

There is overwhelming clinical research to substantiate the *in*validity of skin testing to diagnose food allergy, yet I do not know of one allergist who doesn't bill insurance companies for these inaccurate tests. Allergists have long fought blood tests for food allergies. This is because food immune responses are most likely due to the formation of different antibodies (a white blood cell's response to anything foreign in the blood stream – like a pollen) than airborne allergy and these can not be detected on skin tests.

Skin testing can only determine one type of allergic response, which is rarely food induced. It is sad that the well being of the public is often disregarded when finances are at stake. It seems that much of the medical profession just doesn't appear to care about the truth. The mentality seems to be, "If a doctor orders a test, he must be right." Be careful out there!

This chapter will counsel you on trying to naturally relieve both inhalant allergies and food allergies. After all, do you really

want to know what you're allergic to, or do you want relief?
My friends, if we dare to overcome our allergies by ourselves,
then we also dare to overcome our allergists by ourselves.

Allergies and Fungus

by David A. Holland, M.D.

"I've never had allergies before I moved to Dallas!" the patient tells me as she, or he, speaks with a nasal voice and sniffles.

"How long have you lived here?" I ask.

"About a year and a half, now."

This is a typical scenario I encounter several times a week, and I'm just one guy in one office. I wonder how many other doctors hear this on a weekly basis.

East Texas is the perfect place to develop mold allergies. There is humidity, rain, and the usual winds: perfect for disturbing the mold spores following the rains.

"My allergies get worse when it's raining or when it's humid," is another frequently heard comment.

"Allergies" is a broad topic, and one that we had a difficult time narrowing down. You've got your classic sinus allergies or allergic rhinitis. This is also called "hay fever" and is accompanied by symptoms of sneezing, watery eyes, runny nose, etc. You've got allergies to drugs like penicillin (which, as you know by now, is a mold by-product). Then you've got

133

asthma, skin allergies like hives and eczema – the list goes on and on. "Hay fever," by the way, was a term derived from the manifestation of fever after being exposed to *Aspergillus*-laden, moldy hay. So you can already begin to see how fungus is inevitably tied into allergies!

Obviously we want to discuss further how fungus can be related to why you feel so miserable. Grab that box of Aloe Vera Puffs before you start. OK, now – read on!

Dr. C. Orian Truss, M.D., an early pioneer in the work and study of candidiasis and its relation to various illness and symptom patterns, describes "the familiar manifestations of allergy" related to exposure to and infestation with the *Candida albicans* yeast. *Candida albicans* is one of the most allergic substances known and studied. See Dr. Truss's book *The Missing Diagnosis* published in 1985 and his article, "Tissue Injury Induced by Candida albicans," in the appendix of his book. Dr. Truss continues: "Once the mucous membranes become inflamed by their allergic response to yeast products, infection begins to occur with great regularity at random sites from the nose to the lungs."

Patients often come into the doctor's office not so much because of allergies but because of the subsequent infections that they cause due to the chronic congestion in the sinuses and lungs. At this point, antibiotics and possibly steroids are prescribed, both of which lead to further stimulation of fungal and yeast growth. Do you see how a vicious cycle can be created at this point?

R. J. Hay, in "Fungal Infections" (*Manson's Tropical Diseases.* Cook, G. C. W. B. Saunders, Inc. 1996. Chapter 59), informs us that hay fever or asthma due to molds like *Aspergillus*, *Alternaria*, and *Penicillium* species is estimated to account for *up to 15%* of respiratory allergies! That means one in six of you with hay fever may actually be infested with a mold that is causing your allergic symptoms. And you thought it was just because allergies run in your family!

An article in *Chest* (Adjunctive Therapy of Allergic Broncho-pulmonary Aspergillosis with Itraconazole. Denning, David W., et. al. September, 1991. 100:3.) describes how **100%** of patients with severe asthma symptoms due to *Aspergillus* fungus experienced improvement in symptoms after being treated with an *antifungal* medicine called Sporanox, or Itraconazole.

How do you know if your symptoms of allergy or asthma are due to a fungus? You might consider trying an antifungal program with a changed diet and antifungal remedies and see if you don't feel much better. Your other option is to live an occasionally miserable, and sometimes life-threatening, exist-ence. Analyze what you might lose by trying the former. This is what Doug is talking about when he refers to "branching out" and educating yourself on your disease.

How about those of you with hay fever, allergies, or asthma in your childhood but you "grew out of it?" It is known that "sensitization to fungi is high in childhood and declines rapidly with age" (*American Journal of Respiratory Critical Care*

Medicine. June 1996. 6:151:2109-2115.). If you continue to have allergies as an adult, you can almost be certain that you are still having problems with fungi. I am convinced that childhood asthma has very little to do with genetics, dirty carpets, and cockroaches and more to do with diet, antibiotics, and molds.

I think that people with hay fever want to know if there is any hope and if there really is a "magic bullet" to rid them of their miseries. I can only speak of the number of people who walked into Doug's office with Kleenex in their hands, wiping their noses, and two weeks later were using the Kleenex for tears of joy because their life-long miseries were on the way *out* of their lives. Granted, none of those who did not put forth an effort shared in the joy. Changing the way you live and eat is no easy feat. But neither is living a life with allergies.

I am no allergist and have no interest in becoming one. I do expect some criticism in, perhaps, lack of scientific evidence of molds being linked to most cases of allergies. But once you piece together the literature that *is* out there and know the right questions to ask your patients, it is evident that molds cause more allergies and asthma problems than a physician would ever imagine. And I doubt that I could ever convince the American Academy of Allergy, Asthma, and Immunology, which is a large and powerful group of specialty doctors. So, I'll continue to let the patients tell their own stories. You just can't argue with results!

What I'd Do ...

by Doug A. Kaufmann

If you carefully read Dr. Holland's section, "Allergies and Fungus," you know that logic sometimes supercedes science. I believe that unless you dig for many months you will not find a plethora of scientific literature implicating fungus as causing allergy and asthma. But neither will you find a scientific link to sugar causing hyperactivity, even though parents know this is the case. Scientists can often be very careful to hide truths that may injure their credibility or income. Unfortunately, this may be the case in dealing with allergy.

Like all diseases in America, allergy is a progressive problem – it's getting worse every year. Specialists, called allergists, struggle to understand this mysterious disease and the intricacies of an immune system that would allow seemingly harmless antigens, like cedar or elm pollen, cat hair/dander, or wheat, to create such havoc.

If I suffered from allergies, I'd probably find an *immunologist* at the local medical school who would help me to better understand my condition. Immunologists are not medical doctors; rather, they are immune system researchers. They receive doctor of philosophy degrees in immunity and are quite knowledgeable about allergies. I'd also try to find an ear, nose, and throat allergist as opposed to a regular allergist. ENT

doctors, in my opinion, have a superior testing system (the
Rinkle Serial Dilution System) and are more in tune to foods
and fungus being the causes of allergies. I am of the opinion
that foods and fungus are far more important to understand than
are dust and pollen. You can often control food and fungus
yourself! Turning your allergies over to a nurse giving two to
three shots weekly means losing control over your condition.
And you thought insurance companies really had *your* best
interest at heart!

Based on my knowledge of allergy and immunology, if I
suffered from allergies, here's what I would do:

First, I would get to a doctor and have a <u>Total IgE</u> blood test.
Although a family doctor may run this test for you, I've found
that allergists may not want to run this test. You see, the results
of this simple, inexpensive blood test may cost an allergist
hundreds of dollars in skin tests. Protective protein immuno-
globulins (also known as antibodies) come in five classes. One
of them, *immunoglobulin E*, known as the allergy antibody,
normally runs from 0 – 150 in healthy, non-allergic adults. The
problem for any allergist is that many of his patients who
appear allergic have very normal levels of this immunoglobulin. Instead of trying to figure out this discrepancy, allergists
often exclude the use of this blood test.

Please allow me to interject my limited knowledge regarding
this blood test. It is my assertion that *most* people who appear
to be allergic actually have either post-therapeutic dysbiosis
(intestinal overgrowth of fungus or bad bacteria provoking

allergies following antibiotics or other medicines) or mold allergy that will not elevate the level of IgE in their blood. In either case, allergy tests need not be done – in my humble opinion. Rather, I'd follow the recommendation listed below if my Total IgE was within the normal range.

Next, I'd change my diet to preclude fungal and mold growth. Most environmental fungi are saprophytic, meaning they consume dead and decaying material. Once inside the human body, however, they become parasitic – they require a host (that's us, kids) for food supply. They love yeast (baker's and brewer's) and sugar. They are not particular as to what form the sugar comes in, so fruits (fructose), table sugar (sucrose), all grains, breads, pastas, beans, and potatoes should be avoided due to their carbohydrate content.

If I had nasal sinus allergies, I'd use a nasal spray made from grapefruit extract such as NutriBiotic's "Grapefruit Nasal Spray." Grapefruit is quite a good fungicide and often fungi inhabit the nasal pharyngeal passage. This nasal spray costs only about $10 and I'd take two puffs three times daily for a few weeks to see if that helped.

A product made by Solaray called QBC seems to work well for allergic individuals. The "Q" stands for quercitin. This citrus bioflavinoid seems to block the receptor sites on allergy cells, thereby limiting binding of pollens. The "B" stands for bromelain, often used for inflammatory problems, and the "C" stands for vitamin C.

Herbs, used by people for centuries, seem to be specific to each individual case of allergy. Whereas one person can take *Eyebright* for eye allergies and have great results, another may have no results whatsoever. This can be logically explained by the toxicity threshold of each individual. A very toxic individual may have to detoxify prior to worrying about their allergies.

It is my opinion that one day science will find that literally any seed that survives the germination process is an antifungal. Fungus is so prevalent in soil that it engulfs and consumes many plant seeds. Those that it doesn't consume could become vigilant fungicides. Today, scientists have studied onion, garlic, and grapefruit, to name a few, and have found that these have fungicidal effects. Just imagine the magnitude of my hypothesis! Any organic food or herb could be used to control allergy, but only if the etiology of the allergy is fungus! Since many pharmaceutical drugs are derived from herbs, one could argue that pharmaceutical medicines work by eliminating fungal proliferation! And guess what? Many do! The point is, you will find numerous herbal remedies for allergic conditions and some sufferers swear by them. Just remember that the reason they work may have more to do with the etiology of a person's allergy (fungus?!) than the herbal remedy, itself.

The ecology of the intestines is crucial, and when this is out of sync (a condition called dysbiosis), allergic reactions can occur. If, for example, you've had horrible allergies since taking birth control pills, steroids, or antibiotics, it is likely that these pills could have altered the terrain of the bowel enough to bring about the allergies. This being the case, I'd try a wonderful product made by Natren[1]. It is called *Healthy Trinity* and is a replacement therapy for the upper and lower intestines. Be careful, because not all good bacterial replacements are the same. Natren has stood the test of time and has very high quality ingredients.

When it is difficult to establish a basis for your misery, try increasing the productivity of your immune system. This is assisted with a nutrient called *Beta-Glucans*. The Seagate Company in San Diego has an excellent beta-glucans, which they mix with either organic carrot powder or pure shark cartilage. The NSC Company in Reno, Nevada also has an excellent beta-glucans called either NSC100 or NSC24. Long published...

I know that my frustration with the medical community can be discerned in my writings, but there really are doctors like David Holland out there. Many actually take an interest in their patients' struggles and are happy to learn that something other than traditional allergy tests and shots work for their patients. Most doctors, other than allergists, know that traditional allergy work-ups and desensitizing injections aren't the answer. Otherwise, they would send all of their allergic patients to allergists – something not many doctors do any more.

Most importantly, if you have a good relationship with your doctor, then know the importance of educating him or her as to what controls the allergic symptoms their prescription couldn't control! You'd be surprised how many doctors would welcome a nice letter from a patient informing them that *stinging nettles* relieved their allergies. And, who knows, perhaps his next cure could be thanks to you!

1. See Appendix B for contact information for this and other products mentioned throughout the book.

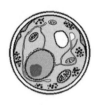

Chapter Nine

Relating Fungus to Women's Health

Women's Yeast-Related Health Problems

by Doug A. Kaufmann

What comes to mind when those two words, "yeast infection," are said? Vaginal yeast, right? This chapter will explore issues deeper than doctors are capable of! By the time you put this book down, you will likely have more knowledge than most physicians as to the significance of those two seemingly harmless words, "yeast infection."

Perhaps not all female health problems are generated by yeast or fungus, but once a determination has been made that a fungus is the cause of a woman's health disorder, inevitably the question as to how the microorganism entered her body should be explored. This can actually occur in many ways.

Once the fungal spores gain access, they can disseminate throughout the body quite easily via the bloodstream. Inhalation of fungal spores creates one portal of entry and often mimics asthma or any number of respiratory diseases. Sexual transmission of fungal spores is known to exist, as will be discussed later in this chapter. I believe, as do many other health professionals, that most fungal infections directly involve the use of broad-spectrum antibiotics. In my opinion, one of the first questions any medical practitioner should ask his patients is whether *any* symptoms began shortly after taking *any* antibiotic, thereby helping to confirm a cause and effect relationship. Although many women link vaginal yeast to antibiotics, more complex symptoms could and should be attributed to these medicines. Antibiotics as a cause of yeast infections have been very well documented for decades. Less understood, but of equal importance, is the causal role of hormones in yeast infections. Prescriptive hormones include steroids, such as cortisone, prednisone, and the birth control pill.

One interesting note, here, is a confirmation of my long-term hypothesis that yeast and fungi are directly linked to cancer. John Glaspy, M.D., medical director of the UCLA Joint Medical-Surgical Oncology Center, recently stated, "Theoretically, *all* hormone treatments/hormone replacement therapy (HRT), birth control pills, and fertility drugs can cause cancer." Since there is good evidence that all steroidal hormones can increase fungal overgrowth, this statement may finally add fuel to the fire of the link between cancer and fungi.

I feel compelled to apprise every woman of the fact that we have known for years that fungi can be transmitted sexually (Oriel, J. D., et. al. Genital yeast infections. British Medical Journal. 4:761. 1972). Unfortunately, not much is published about this important phenomenon. Although I have no scientific documentation to confirm this, it appears that male alcohol intake plays a vital role in some female health problems. If I might venture a guess, I'd say that men who drink beer (grain, sugar, and yeast!) maintain a skin fungal condition that can be transmitted during sexual intercourse. These fungi remain dormant on the male exterior dermis, where the temperature is

70 to 80 degrees. Once a 99 degree mucous membrane tissue is involved, they seem to activate and proliferate. In the early stages, a woman might not notice any symptoms. Within a few days or weeks, these fungi may mobilize within the female reproductive tract, causing widespread damage including endometriosis, vaginal yeast, painful intercourse, and bladder infections. Remember when we called bladder infections "honeymoon cystitis?" Why did we know then but not now that female bladder infections were linked to a male partner? Not surprisingly, symptomatic relief often accompanies the use of appropriate prophylactic measures. You can now understand why I believe that men's prostate problems are directly linked to fungi. Fungal prostatitis has been reported in numerous scientific journals. Once fungus has been transplanted to the proper (female) host and becomes activated, the male is vulnerable to infection – not on the skin, as was the case when he was the carrier, but now within the urethra and the male reproductive tract. The urethra of the male passes directly through the prostate, which is exposed during sexual intercourse. In my humble opinion, anything capable of making bread swell just by adding heat and moisture is also capable of making *any* tissue, including the prostate gland, swell just by adding heat and moisture! Testicular pain is also a common complaint, as this yeast is exchanged between sexual partners.

What symptoms can fungi and yeast cause once activated within the female? I believe that the list is endless. Certainly, when one understands the danger of toxins produced by fungi, it is plausible to claim that infertility, miscarriage, painful intercourse, menstrual problems, false positive pap smears, lumps, cysts, and endometriosis, to name a few, could each involve fungi. Think about this fact: prepubescent girls have ovaries and a uterus, yet never have ovarian or uterine cysts or endometriosis! Why is that? A male sexual partner just has to figure in somewhere! Conversely, all boys have a prostate gland, but only men get prostatitis! Why does this fact seem so obvious to you and me, yet allopathic medicine has never even broached the subject?

For the record, I do not believe in mammography. This "business" of finding cancer early presupposes that we even know what cancer is. According to John Lee, M.D., since 1992, most pathologists have known that *"carcinoma" in-situ* duct cells *do not* progress to cancerous breast tumors; yet surgery, chemotherapy, and radiation done following this diagnosis create an illusion that mammography really works. I do believe, however, that mammography represents a very accurate breast fungal test. Even calcium oxalate deposits have been identified in tissues infected by some fungi. These truths may be withheld from the general public because of the sizeable business that cancer has become. Even our federal government is involved in the business of cancer: the U.S. Postal Service has released its "Fund the Cure" stamp to help "stamp out" breast cancer: at 40 cents per stamp.

It is abnormal for fungi to live inside the human body. Fungi are ubiquitous in nature and are saprophytic. This means that they survive by ingesting dead or decaying material. Many fungi become parasitic once inside the human body. This fact may account for the dietary cravings that men and women have when suffering from internal yeast and fungal overgrowth. Parasites are alive and must eat. Fungal parasites must have sugar in order to thrive. So often we see people who eat very little, yet are extremely bloated, gaseous, and overweight. Most have numerous intestinal problems, including bloating, belching, gas, constipation, diarrhea, indigestion, or reflux. Ironically, most crave potatoes, pasta, sodas, bread, and sugar. *These are the very foods that fungi must have in order to thrive.* I have long contended that people who have fungal infections really can't control their cravings. They must keep the parasitic fungi fed or risk illness, themselves, as the fungi die!

Allow me to quote one sentence from a respected medical textbook: "That animals may be fattened on a predominantly carbohydrate diet demonstrates the ease of conversion of carbohydrate into fat." Yet again, nutritional myths of calorie counting or low-fat diets contributing to weight loss are exposed! Although this may be the case in some weight loss, it is certainly not the case in all. Ladies, it is very likely that if you have an internal fungal condition, the few foods you are eating are precisely the wrong ones. What about vegetarian diets? Remember, that fungi love tofu, breads, beans, and rice, but don't like meat. So many women that we counsel tell us that they eat a healthy vegetarian diet but feel miserable. I simply ask, "Healthy for whom?" Are *you* thriving, or is the fungus inside of you thriving?

You are probably tired of hearing me say, "Why hasn't any medical school or research organization resolved what seems so logical to you and me?" To solve this puzzle, simply travel

149

50 years back in time with me. Didn't four out of five doctors smoke Camels in 1948? Didn't we respect doctors enough to know that since they were medically trained, they *must* know what was necessary for optimum health?! Now this same profession is involved in litigation with the cigarette industry for something that their peers actively condoned a few decades ago! Was the past generation of physicians duped into believing that sucking on sugar-dipped tobacco leaves was really good for health; or did the tobacco industry literally buy their support from the American Medical Association?

Today, folks, it is likely that four out of five doctors prescribe antibiotics for their family members and their patients. No, doctors don't smoke any more; but you must understand that today medical schools receive millions of dollars in financial assistance not from the tobacco industry, but, rather, from the pharmaceutical industry. Where, then, are the medical institutions' loyalties today? Please think about this the next time you are handed a prescription following a brief medical exam. Is this really the best thing you can do for your medical condition, or was your doctor's medical training biased?

On the subject of yeast problems and women, David Holland, M. D., will give us his take on this interesting subject. Richard Mabray, M.D., a prominent gynecologist, has gained quite a reputation in medicine for his intense studies and research into the role of yeast and fungi in female health problems. You'll find Dr. Mabray's article very supportive of what you have really known all along: that yeast and fungi can cause debilitating medical symptoms.

When we finally comprehend the biases involved and the negative impact that many pharmaceutical drugs have had on our health, the field of medicine will begin to change. I'm certain that the power of an aroused public will have an impact on the very industry that *received* millions of dollars of very questionable grants and gifts, just as it did 50 years ago.

Women and Fungi
Not the description of a successful date!

by David A. Holland, M.D.

"Study ties cases of vaginal thrush
to baker's yeast! The yeast was apparently
transferred from hand to vagina."

Medical Tribune, June 5, 1997

As ridiculous as the second statement above sounds, it is the
general consensus, or misunderstanding and ignorance, of the
health care field as to the etiology of certain illnesses which,
upon closer inspection, can usually be linked directly to a yeast
or fungus. The researchers may not have known of a study
published 20 years earlier in the *Journal of the American
Medical Association* (JAMA) where Mary Miles, M. D., et. al.,
discovered in 1977 that 100 percent of women with vaginal
yeast had the same yeast isolated from their stool. They
concluded that eradication of chronic yeast infections would be
impossible without prior eradication of the gut yeast. In other
words, the individuals in the study listed above probably
contracted the vaginal yeast from *eating* the yeast bread! This
has been questioned subsequently, however, because women
can still become infested with vaginal yeast despite having
negative stool cultures (C. C. Kibbler).

Why do we get these infections? I believe the answer lies in
one's diet, or the *wrong* diet I should say. Again, this is just me
going out on a limb, but there is some rather compelling
evidence that this may be true.

153

As you may recall, many fungi produce poisons called mycotoxins that can adversely affect the fungal host (the human
body, in this case). Most mycotoxins suppress the immune
system. They interfere with its normal function. In fact, we
take advantage of this when we give kidney transplant recipi-
ents the mycotoxin called cyclosporine. Yes, this drug is a
mycotoxin. Cyclosporine essentially shuts down our immune
system so that the body will not reject the new kidney, which is
basically a foreign object in the recipient's body. Our immune
system is designed to reject foreign substances, but this reaction is not desirable in the case of a transplant. The negative
aspect of immune suppression is that we are now left vulnerable to attack by *any* invading critter, namely fungal, bacterial,
and viral organisms. If your immune system does not work,
you will continue to get sick!

Let's say that we are not taking the drug cyclosporine, which
should be the case unless you just received a new kidney. How,
then, can my immune system be suppressed by these fungal
poisons, you might ask. The answer, again, may lie in your
diet. Stored grains that become moldy are introduced either
into the grain portion of your diet or your meats by way of
cows and pigs being fed moldy grains. The FDA has established limits regarding the amount of *some* of the mycotoxins
allowed in foods. Other potentially dangerous mycotoxins
have had no limitations placed on them. Mycotoxins and
molds are an insurmountable problem for farmers and can
result in huge losses. For example, between 1977 and 1981
about one-third of the milled corn from the southeast U. S.
contained levels of *aflatoxin* that were too high for human

consumption (Mycotoxins, Economic and Health Risks. Task Force Report. No. 116. November 1989. Council for Agricultural Science and Technology – CAST). So where did that moldy corn go? It was diverted away from our table into cattle feed! So even if we aren't consuming the contaminated grain directly, we may get chronic low levels in the fat of our meat (thus, trimming the fat may be useful for this reason and this only).

Some of these toxins, like *aflatoxin*, have been linked to cancers and atherosclerosis; but our interest for this chapter is in the role these toxins may play in female diseases. This is an interest of mine, as well. How many women do you hear of undergoing a hysterectomy due to fibroids? Or how many are getting breast biopsies because of a nodule they found? Or who doesn't know of someone who is having trouble getting pregnant, or even having trouble remaining pregnant? If a female is given high doses of the hormone *estrogen*, a number of atypical health events may take place including growth of the uterus and the breasts (could this *cause* cancer?). It would also be difficult for her to have a normal pregnancy because normal estrogen-progesterone ratios are needed by the body to both enable and maintain a pregnancy.

Let's say that you don't give her estrogen, but something that mimics it. A mycotoxin called zearalenone would fit that role. Interestingly, zearalenone is a mycotoxin found primarily in corn and corn-based products, such as cereal and corn meal, as well as in bananas world wide. It may also be a residue in the meat of cattle consuming contaminated corn (Mycotoxins.

CAST.) Zearalenone is produced by a mold called *Fusarium graminearum*, which can invade and grow on corn in the field or in storage bins. Of interest is that zearalenone in cattle and swine has been associated with infertility and can interfere with fetal development, ovulation, conception, and viability of newborn animals. It can cause swelling of mammary glands and feminization of young male swine. The toxin mimics the effect of the hormone estrogen, and can have effects in concentrations as minute as one part per million!

What is being done to protect you against this toxin? The true answer is, "I don't know." While there are recommendations and enforced levels for a few mycotoxins, there are currently *no* limits or recommended levels of zearalenone placed on foods and grains for human consumption (Charles Wobshuk. Department of Botany and Plant Pathology. Purdue University). To have a zero-tolerance for these toxins would be cost-prohibitive; we just have to do the best we can.

As important as it is to uncover the fact that these problems exist in our food supply, of even greater importance is admitting they may be contributing to some chronic health problems. I would exercise caution with food choices. If you already have a weakened immune system or are chronically ill, then I'd change my diet and get that immune system working again. See the diet in the appendix for more information on this subject.

Maintaining the Delicate Balance

by C. R. Mabray, M.D.

Yeast infections and problems are so common that everyone,
both healers and patients, know about them. And that's a
problem! Most patients and nearly all physicians think of
vaginal and vulvar itching, irritation, and discharge as all there
is to a yeast "infection." Therefore, it simply does not compute
that abnormal nail growth, scalding under the arms, acne, red
rash around the mouth and nose, fatigue, joint pain, tendonitis,
diarrhea, constipation, liver stress, etc. may all be symptoms of
a yeast problem.

We have been brought up in a medical culture where we
identify an offending germ or agent, find some drug to kill that
offender, and then get "well." The problem is just not that
simple. For many, if not most, the problem is an immune
sensitivity to the yeast or a reaction to one of the scores of
poisons or toxins that these yeasts are capable of producing. It
is not always a simple infection. In fact, those with uncompli-
cated genital infections are the easiest to treat.

First, let me illustrate the immune aspect. We have poison ivy
in our back yard from time to time. I can handle it with my
bare hands and suffer no ill effect, whereas my son is so
sensitive that he will suffer just being nearby while I cut and
move the plant. He is "allergic" to poison ivy. In like manner,

those having the most symptomatic and most treatment-resistant yeast problems are sensitive or "allergic" to the organism or to the toxins produced by the organism. Moreover, there is a close kin to other fungi, and folks most sensitive to candida yeasts almost always have heightened sensitivity to other yeasts, fungi, and molds. Thus, we must contend with one's total internal and external environment in order to get best treatment results. For example, if your house has been flooded and there is a fungal/mold growth in the walls or air-conditioning ducts or under the carpet, simply treating your yeast infection will neither restore nor maintain wellness. You must address the total load on your defense system.

Another significant problem with molds is their toxin production. Just the candida species, alone, has been demonstrated to have nearly 100 distinctly different powerful toxins (poisons) that have specific impact on the human body. Some attack nervous tissue, some attack muscle, others attack connective tissues such as bone and joint tissue. Therefore, symptoms may vary dramatically depending upon the toxin produced, the target organ affected, and the integrity of our defense capabilities.

Bear in mind that "yeasts" are really not the problem. They are here on earth to be garbage recycling factories. If dead organisms were not recycled, the earth would cease to be habitable – dead things would just pile up to the moon. Converting dead organisms to a useable form requires the powerful chemical secretions of yeasts, mold, fungi, and bacteria which are capable of transforming once-living organisms into "dirt."

The process of life may begin again through the miracle of photosynthesis, which is the basis of our whole food chain and existence. These toxins must be powerful to do their job. They are meant to be a blessing. It is only when the system gets out of balance inside our bodies through stress, antibiotic exposure, high-sugar diet, injury, chemical exposure, etc. that the toxins become our enemy rather than our friend.

In summary, yeast problems vary from easy and straightforward to complex and convoluted. Symptoms may occur because of infection, sensitivity (allergy), toxin exposure, or some combination. These symptoms seldom exist without an imbalance in your personal eco-life-health system.

Successful defeat of symptoms may involve simple changes of lifestyle and environment, or may respond only to drastic adjustments, plus supplements, plus allergy management, plus medication. In either case, be prepared to take control of your own life and health – that's the only way it works well!

Chapter Ten

Relating Fungus to Pain

The Ability of Fungus to Cause Pain

by Doug A. Kaufmann

According to the book *Alternative Medicine*[1], chronic pain has become the United States' most common health disorder affecting nearly one in three Americans and costing nearly 40 billion dollars a year in bills and lost wages. With another one in three of us suffering from heart disease and another one in three suffering from cancer, well, you get the picture. That which isn't killing us is hurting us!

My own back pain became so unbearable in my early 20s that my roommates jokingly rigged up a pulley over my bed to assist me in getting up each morning. There were actually days I wished it were functional, because I would have used it! Twenty-eight years later, although I have had intermittent flare-ups on rare occasions, my back pain is gone. Most importantly, I know exactly how to exacerbate this horrible pain. Why is that so important? Well, if you know how to provoke pain, then you also know how to subdue it. Ironically, when I consume too much sugar, my back pain is upon me like white on rice. If I dare sleep in the wrong position or lift anything the day after a sugar binge, you can bet money that I'll be out of commission for a few days. Logic might dictate, therefore, that as the breadwinner in my family, I avoid sugar and, therefore, avoid lost time at work. The combination of being self-employed and breadwinner is especially tough because when I

163

don't work, we don't eat. As a quick learner, I carefully choose my down time. I happen to love mom's fudge at Christmas time. I take two weeks off at year's end for a totally different reason than most people: recuperation!

Pain is so common that ten years ago a prominent headache specialist wrote a book educating physicians on the proper methods of encoding insurance forms for payment when dealing with headaches. Entitled *Headache Classification System, A Diagnostic Code Manual*, this book contains 376 pages. Mind you, this is only headache pain! Just imagine the diagnostic book for back pain! I had a chiropractic friend who had a giant book which listed the causes of subluxation (a dislocation of a joint, so that the bone ends are misaligned but still in contact) and general back pain. Lifting the book was listed on page 945! The point is, there are as many causes of pain as there are people with pain. Neither of these books on back or headache pain listed sugar or fungus as etiologic factors, but they sure do provoke my back pain! Sugars feed parasitic fungus. Like many things in medicine, these books prove that the simplest concepts are often the last to be accepted.

Those who suffer from pain tend to be their own best doctors. I have always believed that the best orthopedic physicians in the world would be those who suffered from pain. You can bet that these physicians have employed techniques in their practices additional to what medical school taught them. Life experiences often provide better lessons than books.

You know that I believe that fungus, either acting alone or in unison with its metabolites, causes nearly every malady known to man. The two leading causes of death in the United States are heart disease and cancer. There is reason to believe that we remain ignorant as to why these diseases are killing so many because the medical profession has not been properly educated in the field of mycology, the study of fungi.

We have expounded upon both the physical symptoms caused by fungi and the impact of fungi on the brain and nervous system. As you may recall, several respected scientific authors have concluded that fungi, once inside the human body, are known to disseminate. This spreading of fungi can lead to tissue impregnation and affect tissues and organs far from the original portal of entry. The portal of entry can be respiratory, via inhalation of spores, can be the skin, via puncture or transdermal entrance, can be ingesting it through what we eat, or can be the end result of sexual contact with a person that has a localized fungal disease in the genitalia.

Once parasitic fungi have found a new host, numerous symptoms and diseases can be initiated but not always immediately. I happen to believe that in most healthy individuals, although dissemination can occur quickly, pain and suffering caused by these fungi may take decades. For this reason, do not ever underestimate the fact that your pain may be linked with a slow growing, insidious pathogen. If this were the case, what preexisting conditions would have led to the subjective symptoms, called pain, that you now suffer from?

As I mentioned earlier, my pain is directly linked with sugar. Ironically, the pain does not exacerbate upon eating sugar on each occurrence. I might not experience any pain associated with eating a bowl of ice cream. If I stop there, I'm fine! I still feel, however, that I have this underlying addiction to sugar. So the harmless bowl of ice cream becomes a bowl of pasta the following evening, followed by a dessert that I rarely eat. Soon, I'm finding it impossible to avoid potatoes, excessive fruits, and even chocolate. Before this addiction has ended, you can bet that during my daily routine I'll twist the wrong way and, BINGO, the pain begins. The difference in your pain and my pain is that, during the past 25 years, I've been able to trace mine directly to increased carbohydrate consumption. It is my contention that nine in ten of you would be able to discover the etiology of your pain given enough time and a sincere interest in the root cause, thereby leading to recovery. After reading this chapter, you may want to take steps enabling you to not only discover the roots of your pain, but also to eliminate it!

1. Burton Goldberg Group. *Alternative Medicine: The definitive guide.* 1995. Future Medicine Publishing, Inc. Fife, Washington.

Fibromyalgia and Chronic Fatigue Syndrome

by David A. Holland, M.D.

Definitions

Fibromyalgia (FM) – a disorder of *unknown etiology* characterized by, among many other symptoms, fatigue, musculoskeletal pain, and muscle stiffness   (*Harrison's Principles of Internal Medicine.* 12th Ed. 1991.)

Chronic fatigue syndrome (CFS) – also of *unknown etiology*, is currently diagnosed by the occurrence of:

➤New onset fatigue of greater than six month duration with a 50 percent decrease in normal activity

➤No other medical or psychiatric conditions that could explain the symptoms

➤Six to eight of the following symptoms and at least two physical signs (unless you have all eight symptoms). Symptoms: low grade fever, sore throat, painful lymph node swelling, generalized muscle weakness, muscle aches, headaches, migratory joint aches, and sleep disturbances; Signs: body temperature of 37.5–38.6 degrees C, pharyngitis, or palpable cervical or axillary lymph node swelling (*Griffith's Five-Minute Clinical Consultant.* 1991.)

167

You might have CFS by now from just reading the list! Never mind technicalities; these are used for diagnostic purposes. If you have been diagnosed with FM or CFS, then once you get past the medical jargon, all you really care about is that you feel BAD and you want to know what you can do to feel GOOD!

I looked up CFS on the internet and came up with over 100,000 sites to search through. I quit after reviewing a hundred or so, because it soon became clear that no one was coming up with any definite answers regarding these elusive disorders, although there are a lot of unproven theories.

In this section we are discussing what we believe based on clinical observation to be the etiology of CFS and FM. In addition, although CFS and FM are two separate disorders, they share many common symptoms and will, therefore, be considered together in this discussion.

Myalgic encephalomyelitis, a term introduced in 1957 in the United Kingdom, is what we know today in the United States as chronic fatigue syndrome (Scand, J. Work Environment Health. Suppl. 23. 1997. 3:17-34). The timing of the appearance of this "disorder" is interesting in that antibiotic use was becoming more prevalent at the time, having recently been introduced as the new "magic bullet" for bacterial infections. One might wonder if the timing is more than coincidence, since it is well known that antibiotic use is a risk factor for yeast and fungal overgrowth (Kibbler, C. C. *Principles and Practice of Clinical Mycology*. 1996. Pg. 9).

Is there any proof that fungi and yeast cause FM or CFS? None, directly, that I came across. However, one must examine cause and effect and consider what treatments have worked to retrospectively diagnose what must have been the cause. I have seen, time and time again, clients initiate an anti-fungal/anti-mycotoxin diet and take anti-fungal medications in an attempt to rid themselves of their fatigue, only to have complete and long term success and recovery. *If the successful treatment was anti-fungal, then the cause was fungal*!

It has been said that no amount of negative studies can offset one single positive clinical observation. In addition, it would be difficult to isolate the causative fungus in any situation to prove a link, since *"dissemination of yeasts is unlikely to be recognized because they are rarely identified ... in the routine laboratory."* (Kibbler, C. C.) Our medical laboratories are simply not adept at routinely isolating fungi from human tissue or fluid samples.

I did come across one study (*Medical Hypotheses*. June, 1995. 44[6]:507-515) describing the fact that patients with "chronic candidiasis syndrome" shared many of the same symptoms as those with CFS. It also mentioned that patients with CFS had improvement in their symptoms after taking oral anti-fungal medication. Lastly, the study acknowledged the fact that patients with candida overgrowth (as in chronic mucocutaneous candidiasis) had suppression in their cellular immunity, a finding also seen in CFS patients. Without an intact cellular immune system, one is susceptible to reactivation of such viral infections as shingles, herpes zoster, and Epstein-Barr virus

(EBV). Thus, in cases of CFS that were suspected to be *caused* by EBV, one can now see that the true initiating factor of the fatigue was the fungal overgrowth, or more rightly so, the factor *that caused the fungal overgrowth*, whether it be antibiotics, birth control pills, etc.

A chapter in *Mycotoxins: Economic and Health Risks* (CAST Task Force Report No. 116. November, 1989. Phone 515-292-2125) discusses in extensive detail the means by which several common mycotoxins impair the immune system. Without an immune system that works, it is inevitable that one will remain chronically ill and susceptible to secondary viral, fungal, and bacterial infections as long as one is exposed to the source of these toxins. Remember, fungi are ubiquitous – they are every where! Again, these toxins may be antibiotics or other mycotoxins that can be found in moldy grains or in moldy-grain-fed animals.

Thus, once again, we have two conditions that have *enormous* economic impacts in terms of lost productivity, diagnosis, and treatment, and, yet, no real answers in the medical field to offer these patients. The huge success with the approaches mentioned above should at very least behoove the medical community to take a closer look into these so-called "alternative" approaches to treatment. This is especially true given the fact that prescriptive medicines like hormones and antibiotics used to treat patients may, in fact, be contributing to the cause of FM and CFS! Having seen the anti-fungal/anti-mycotoxin diet approach work, I am thoroughly convinced that in most, if not all, cases, there is a fungal etiology to FM and CFS.

Craniosacral Manipulation Therapy
What to Do if Your Pain does not Respond
to Food or Fungal Treatment

by Richard Becker, D.O.

As an osteopathic physician, I have come to respect the body's ability to heal itself when given the opportunity to do so. The nerves that control our organs and systemic reactions all come through and around our spine. If the spine is not free to engage full range of motion, pain often ensues. Pain is not the only down side to this condition. A nervous reflex can inhibit healthy organ function which, in turn, can result in disease.

Craniosacral manipulation therapy (CMT) is a form of hands-on physical medicine aimed at correcting the spinal misalignments. Manual manipulation of basic physiologic processes can restore the integrity of the spinal pathways thereby relieving the tissues of pressure they have assumed with the misalignment. As you know, tissues of the body have circulation, otherwise stagnation will occur. The heart consistently pumps blood through the blood vessels. Cerebrospinal fluid (CSF), however, does not have a pumping mechanism to cause circulation. So, just how does the CSF circulate? One chamber of the brain houses the choroid plexus. This plexus actually produces CSF. Tiny, thin layers surrounding the brain and the spinal chord called *meninges* contain small, finger-like projections called *arachnoid villae*. These tiny structures reabsorb CSF. Unlike the constant pumping of the heart to circulate blood, these two CSF processes do not occur simultaneously. Rather, they ebb and flow like the waves in the ocean. In doing so, a pressure wave is created throughout the human body. Skilled osteopathic physicians can literally feel this pulse inside the body and determine blockages. When the spine or internal organs are damaged or diseased, the pressure wave is inhibited. A small amount of pressure (5 – 10 grams), succinctly placed, will completely stop this vital flow of cerebrospinal fluid. By holding the spinal column in a corrupted position, away from the muscle and connective tissue tension, there will be neurologic influences stimulated, thereby restoring proper alignment and active cranial rhythm. Proper blood flow, essential to health, is also restored.

Sounds great, doesn't it? Best of all, it really works! It takes many years of training to perfect this method of treatment, and each therapeutic session requires 30 to 60 minutes to perform. As Doug has told you before, most physicians see 40 to 50 patients daily and could not, therefore, perform such treatments for their patients. This is unfortunate for both the practitioner as well as their patients.

Craniosacral therapy has been proven to help a wide variety of disorders, including arthritis, chronic joint pain, traumatic injuries, bursitis, tendonitis, and a variety of internal organ conditions previously thought to respond only to medications. If you are suffering from ongoing pain, or would simply like to "jump start" your nerves and muscles to good health, consider craniosacral manipulation therapy. It is safe, natural, and, most importantly, it's effective!

Prolotherapy

by Doug A. Kaufmann

Pastor Peter did not survive his deadly cancer. After his death, his close friend, Dr. Ross Hauser, and I stayed in touch with one another, communicating over the fax machine several times weekly. Dr. Hauser is a highly specialized pain therapist called a physiatrist (pron. *fizzy-a-trist*). Such credentials require a graduate medical degree and then an additional four years of residency. There are approximately 5,000 physiatrists in the United States, but only one Ross Hauser. Ross puts the "gentle" in gentleman. His wife, Marion, is the perfect addition to his hectic life. Get these two alone and you'll fully comprehend the opening admonition in his book that you need to lighten up and laugh more often!

Like Dr. Richard Becker, Dr. Hauser's therapy requires the highly skilled brain and hands of a physician. Don't try this on yourself at home! Dr. Hauser performs a therapy called "prolotherapy." This therapy stimulates the areas of pain by inducing an inflammation at the site of pain or injury. This is accomplished by using very thin-gauged needles to direct the natural medicines in the syringe to a specific site. A small amount of the formula is then injected, and several sites surrounding the injury are also injected. It is not uncommon to have Dr. Hauser inject 20 to 50 times during one visit. Since the injections contain a numbing ingredient, this is not as painful as it sounds.

Several visits are often required to terminate the pain, but many people claim to have significant relief following the initial visit. As is the case with Dr. Becker's craniosacral therapy, a variety of pain conditions, including arthritis, back pain, migraine headaches, fibromyalgia, sports injuries, TMJ, herniated discs, and sciatica have all responded favorably to prolotherapy.

Dr. Ross and Marion reduced their knowledge to book form a few years ago. This remarkable book, entitled *Prolo Your Pain Away*, has been so successful that a sequel is forthcoming. The new book will expound on sports injuries and the ability of prolotherapy to cure these.

Yes, I said cure. Why is it that this has become the "four letter word" in clinical medicine? Simply put, the Wall Street beauties of conventional medicine (i.e., pharmaceutical drugs) don't cure anything but the overgrowth of bacteria – and even that returns! They certainly can't cure depression, Alzheimer's disease, or even pain! Despite this, their sales figure are impressive, a clear indication that we prefer adding annuities to the pharmaceutical coffers over investigating breakthrough technologies like prolotherapy.

If you do decide to investigate, don't be surprised if your orthopedic physician gives you the cold shoulder. Do you remember the name that is used for anything that competes with organized medicine? The technology is called "quackery," while the therapists are called "quacks." Based on everything I've learned about honesty and integrity in medicine, I am left wondering who the real "quacks" are!

I have witnessed Dr. Hauser at work on several occasions and have had the opportunity to interview the patients he has performed prolotherapy on. All of the patients I witnessed receiving prolo are thankful and thrilled with the therapy. If your pain is chronic and unrelenting, please consider a hands-on approach – not hands-on a prescription pad, but hands on you!

APPENDIX A

The Initial Phase Diet
by
Doug Kaufmann

The Program

Explanation for Fungal Therapies

Localized or systemic (throughout the body) mycoses (fungi) are not rare. As a matter of fact, they were once commonly and openly referred to within scientific literature as quite common. However, the popularity of bacteria and viruses eventually overshadowed the field of mycology (the study of fungi) and fungi were pushed to the side. Only recently, with accelerated use of chemotherapy, antibiotics, and steroid therapy, have fungi begun to emerge as a serious cause of human illness. This is because immunosuppressed (weak immune system) or hypoimmune hosts (people) are prey to these opportunistic yeasts. "Opportunistic" means that weakened immunity gives opportunity for a fungal infection to thrive. What we do not seem to realize is that *all* of us exposed to antibiotics, steroids, birth control pills, and polluted air, food, and water are likely immunocompromised to some degree.

Fungi can be treated with the use of pharmaceutical drugs or natural remedies depending upon the severity of the infection. Although both remedies seem to work well, drugs sometimes work more quickly. Depending on the type of fungi, a physician may prescribe Nystatin, Lamisil, Nizoral, Diflucan, or Sporanox. Each of these is a prescriptive medicine and each has published side effects.

If you choose to address a fungal problem with natural remedies, you have literally hundreds of options. Some of the most common are listed in this chapter.

Starve the Fungi!

Our Initial Phase Diet (IPD) defines our approach to ridding the body of fungal organisms by starving them. Scientific literature has long referred to dietary patterns that allow fungi to proliferate. We know, for example, that sugar fuels the growth pattern for yeast and fungi. Considering that each American man, woman, and child consumes approximately 130 pounds of sugar annually, it is not surprising that fungi are so difficult to control once they become activated within the human body. Most of us think that the sugars we consume are limited to candy and soda pop. Although our average consumption of soda in America averages 50 gallons yearly per person, our sugar intake is certainly not limited to this type of sugar. Avoiding carbohydrates is also important.

The *Bantam Medical Dictionary* defines carbohydrates as

> ...any one of a large group of compounds including the sugars and starch that contain carbon, hydrogen, and oxygen. Carbohydrates are manufactured by plants and obtained by animals and man from the diet, being one of the three main constituents of food. [Editor's note: protein and fat being the other two.] All carbohydrates are eventually broken down in the body to the simple sugar, glucose, which can then take part in energy-producing metabolic processes.

Carbohydrates are fuel for the body. The fuel is generated by the body's breakdown of certain carbohydrates into sugars. Yet sugar also feeds fungi. Ironically, most of the clients who have fungal disorders consume too much sugar and are exhausted! The right type of carbohydrate in a non-toxic individual will supply energy, however the wrong type of carbohydrate in a fungally-toxic individual actually suppresses energy.

Not only is it important to starve yeasts and fungi, but it is important to avoid and minimize the potent toxins they produce. Vegetables absorb fungal poisons called mycotoxins, carry them out of the body, and inhibit their toxicity. Carotenoids are good chemicals found in vegetables, including xanthophylls, lutein, and lycopene. In one study, carotenoids were found to block the cancer-causing ability of aflatoxin B1 and T2 mycotoxins in experimental animals. Aflatoxin is produced by the mold *Aspergillus* and T2 is made from *Fusarium* mold; both are well known cancer-causing poisons. It has been speculated that the vegetable carotenoids are the very reason vegetables protect against cancer.

Get and Keep the Bowels Moving

It is imperative that, as you kill fungi, they are eliminated from the body. This is a job for the bowels, and too often it is a job poorly done. Non-digestible fiber assists the body in ridding impacted wastes and aids in bowel regularity. The term "non-digestible" means that what goes in must come out, and it will in due time. We specifically recommend psyllium hulls or slippery elm as good sources of this type of fiber. These are available in health food stores and we have found that the powder form is best. Both of these products tend to work best when taken either at the hour of sleep (one tablespoon mixed into water) or divided throughout the day (one heaping teaspoon in water twice daily). It is important to drink plenty of water when taking these forms of fiber. Bottled, spring water, or reverse osmosis water is best. Bulk fibers, such as psyllium hulls and slippery elm, should be used at the discretion of your physician if you have had bowel surgery or a history of intestinal blockage.

If you are constipated and the fiber does not regulate you, you might try cascara sagrada, also obtainable from a health food store. Cascara stimulates peristalsis (moving of the intestines) and should not be taken for long periods of time. Also note that magnesium deficiency can be another cause of constipation.

Repair Oxidative Damage

Free radical molecules are harmful chemicals which can contribute to many symptoms. Skin collagen damage related to free radical injury can be determined with two simple tests.

Do you have a vertical crease in your earlobe? Interestingly, you may be at an increased risk of heart and circulatory damage.

With your hand and arm flat on a table, lift the skin on the back of your hand for a few seconds. Does it snap back when released or does it return to its original dimension slowly? If it returns slowly, this is yet another indication of free radical tissue damage and/or dehydration. If this process occurs on the skin, just imagine what must be going on inside your body!

Proanthocyanidins (PC) are a class of free radical scavengers. You may have heard of two of these PCs, Pycnogenol or grape seed extract. Any health food store has these supplements. At present there is no lab method for determining percentages of OPC (oligomeric proanthocyanidins). Additionally, grape seeds have galic esters, making them more desirable. The usual dosage is approximately one milligram per pound of body weight per day in two or three doses, but it is safe to begin with a larger "loading" dose.

Kill the Fungus!

Only a physician can prescribe a pharmaceutical drug. You, however, may elect to try the following remedies, each of which has antifungal properties. These are available in health food stores, health or organic sections of grocery stores, or nutritionally-oriented pharmacies.

1. **Olive leaf extracts** are antimicrobial agents. Independent lab tests have demonstrated the ability of OLE to eradicate pathogens (any organism capable of causing a disease). OLE contains oleuropein and other active phytochemicals which are responsible for their antimicrobial abilities.

2. **Caprylic acid** is a fatty acid derived from coconut oil. It has potent antifungal properties.

3. **Pau d'arco** is another good antifungal that is either taken in tea form or in capsules. It is the bark of the pau d'arco tree which contains the fungicides. Despite very high humidity in the rain forest, the pau d'arco tree does not grow mold or mildew on its bark.

4. **FORMULA SF722** is actually a brand name (Thorpe Research) for undecalynic acid. Derived from the oil of caster beans, this is another good antifungal product.

5. **Malic acid** is derived from apple cider vinegar and has strong antifungal properties. This can be diluted with water or mixed with fresh-squeezed juice.

6. **Garlic** is one of the most well published antifungals in the world. One of the phyto (plant) enzymes in garlic, **allicin**, is well documented as having anti-microbial properties not limited to the eradication of fungi. It appears viruses and bacteria are also neutralized by garlic. Many supplement companies sell garlic, but since allicin is best used synergistically with other enzymes contained in the garlic, it is best (and most cost effective) to squeeze a clove into your fresh carrot juice.

7. **Carrot juice** contains many important properties, not the least of which inhibits fungal proliferation. A 1988 study in *The Journal of Microbiology* implicated carrot as a good fungus fighter. Again, although the pulp is very important in the carrot, juicing gives your blood stream immediately-available nutrition and gives your digestive juices a break from digesting whole foods.

8. **Tea tree oil**, available in health food stores, seems to work quickly and effectively on local skin fungal problems. Time may prove that anything that survives the germination process in soil has antifungal properties. Fungus would have taken over the world if it were not for antifungal properties in soil. Soil is where certain antifungal drugs (Nystatin) are actually derived. It is important, therefore, to remember the value of organically grown fresh vegetables. Not only are they nutritious, but they may also be antifungal remedies.

Will I be on this diet forever?

No, you will not be on the IPD forever unless you choose to do so. Our Initial Phase Diet (IPD) presents a shock to people. One consolation for you is knowing that each of us working here has been on this diet. We won't ask you to do something we have not done.

Not much is known about fungal diseases because in the 1970s the Center for Disease Control (CDC) decided that fungal diseases were not classified as "notifiable diseases." This means that doctors are not required to report these conditions to regulatory agencies. Hence, a dietary program has never been officially established. The IPD was born out of our under-standing of which foods fed living fungi and which did not. In essence, we are asking you to take the next 14 days to see if you feel better. If you do feel better, this may be due to one of two things: either you have literally starved the living parasitic fungi, microorganisms that must feed on carbohydrates, or you have avoided specific food that you are allergic to. In either case, we will begin experimenting with the reintroduction phase of this program, thereby establishing threshold levels of tolerance to certain carbohydrates and food. Do not be fooled into believing that a 14-day diet will "cure" your fungus problems. We are using this next 14 days to establish whether or not you have a fungal problem and the extent or severity of your condition.

Won't eating eggs and nuts raise my cholesterol?

A great question and one that I asked myself twenty years ago. My experience has been quite the opposite! Blood fats actually reduce while following the IPD. As a matter of fact, fungi produce sterol (cholesterol) and triglycerides. By ridding the body of fungus, blood fats diminish. Recently, studies have confirmed that eggs do not necessarily raise cholesterol after all, and that eating nuts (not peanuts) can even decrease your risk of heart disease by up to 50%!

The general public has been frightened by fat in their diet and often beneficial fats are avoided. Less than one percent of the population actually suffers from a condition where the body cannot handle dietary cholesterol. If you have this rare genetic condition, please speak with your doctor prior to initiating the IPD. Keep in mind that each of us is biochemically unique. The IPD may work wonderfully for one person. It may not work for everyone.

Why should I cook my eggs with the yolk intact?

The combination of oxygen and heat with cholesterol forms *oxysterols*, which are carcinogenic and can induce damage to the lining of the arteries. Unoxidized cholesterol, however, does not have this effect. [See 1. Gary Price Todd, M.D. *Diet, Nutrition, and Disease.* 2. Joseph Hattersley. *Eggs are Great Food!* and 3. *Townsend Letter for Doctors and Patients.* Jan. 1996.] Once you get the eggs on your plate, go ahead and break the yolks!

Isn't eating fat bad for me? Won't I gain weight on the IPD?

There are good fats and bad fats. Eating bad fats is bad, eating good fats is not bad. What are bad fats? Well, margarine and vegetable oils used over and over for deep-frying in restaurants are examples of bad fats. Avocados, raw nuts (except peanuts), eggs, and organic, range-fed meats are all fine. We should, however, note a disclaimer on meats: meat from cattle fed moldy grains (i.e., corn or wheat) is not good. Be careful of restaurant and grocery store meats. The fats of these meats may contain mycotoxins from cattle eating moldy grains.

Have you heard anywhere that meat can cause heart disease and cancer? Mycotoxins are thought to be the reason. Not because of the meat, but because of the dangers associated with our consumption of cattle fed moldy grains. Argentineans consume more beef than any one in the world, yet they have no heart disease or cancer as a result of this. Why? They let their cattle graze in the open fields instead of feeding them moldy grain from silos like we do in the United States.

How will I feel during the program?

Always remember the adage, "No pain, no gain." As we starve yeast and fungi, a phenomenon called "Herxheimer's reaction" may occur. In the 1930s, German dermatologist Dr. Carl Herxheimer first described the body's reaction to the massive killing of microorganisms and the resulting sudden load of toxins released into the blood stream. Also known as "die off," these reactions are typically characterized by flu-like symptoms, chills, aches, and sometimes a low grade fever. It is not rare to suffer from a worsening of the very symptoms you originally experienced. Thirty to forty percent of our clients notice "die off" reactions. This reaction is often a good sign as it verifies that you have been harboring these fungi for quite some time and you have now begun to eradicate them. Like any living thing, they don't like to die! Also, recall that the skin is the largest organ in your body, so it is not rare to see outbreaks or worsening of rashes as the body begins to "clean house." Taking Essiac tea two or three times daily can significantly lessen the Herxheimer's reaction.

How will you know that this is not a reaction to something you are taking? If you are reacting to something that you have just started, you will feel worse and worse. Not so if you are experiencing a "die off" reaction. Within a few days you will feel much better even though you continue taking the supplement. In our experience, the longer the "die off" reaction, the more severe the fungal problem; however, this is not always predictable.

How can I prove that I have a fungal problem?

There are fairly accurate blood tests that detect the presence of antibodies to fungus within the blood stream. One problem with blood tests is that they can detect a past exposure to the fungus; however, they are sometimes inaccurate in picking up present symptoms caused by fungi. Also, by the time these test results are returned to our office, often the client following our program already feels much improvement, thereby ruling out the necessity for the expensive tests. We feel that the best way to confirm that a fungal problem exists is to begin our program and if, within a few days to a few weeks you feel much better, that might be all the confirmation you needed! Also, your response to a fungal questionnaire would be another clue. Often a good medical history tends to support or rule out suspicions of fungal growth.

Is a fungal disorder a "forever" disorder, or can they be successfully eradicated?_____

This is one of the good questions that we are asked every day. Although our IPD and program will not have to be followed forever, please keep in mind that fungi cause diseases. In order to avoid disease, a permanent lifestyle change is necessary.

There are two types of fungal infections. Superficial infections can easily and quickly be remedied. These are conditions like ringworm, jock itch, and vaginal yeast infections. However, fungi can and do impregnate more deeply. These are called "deep mycoses." Depending on how long you have carried the fungus and how deeply it has penetrated, sometimes long-term therapy, including herbal remedies taken by mouth, and diet is necessary. In a 1992 research paper, Orian Truss, M. D., stated that sometimes a two to three year period of treatment is necessary to "clear" the body of fungal poisons. We have confirmed his findings to be true in severe cases. In our experience, if a person had pesticide toxicity in his body or mercury toxicity (especially from mercury amalgam fillings in his teeth), he will clear fungi from his body slowly and be more prone to recurrence of fungi in the future.

Can the Initial Phase Diet (IPD) be dangerous for any one?

Since the IPD is high in proteins, people with advanced kidney disease should be very cautious while on the diet and should work closely with their physicians. In fact, someone with advanced kidney disease should probably avoid this diet since the kidneys may have a problem handling the protein load. The diet, however, will not cause kidney disease in one with healthy kidneys; in fact, it may even prevent kidney disease, according to numerous studies on atherosclerosis (a common cause of kidney damage).

Also, those who are pregnant or breast feeding or who are in childhood years may not be suited to this type of a diet due to the relative reduction of carbohydrates. Those who exercise vigorously may also not do well on a diet that restricts carbohydrates, as these can provide fuel for the body. If you fit into any of these categories, the diet should be discussed with us or your own nutritionist or doctor.

Why should I take psyllium hulls?

Psyllium, being a non-digestible fiber, is one of only three things known to bind fungal poisons (mycotoxins). The other two are charcoal and cholestyramine, a drug. (Costantini, A.V. *Fungalbionics: Cancer*. 1994.) Because psyllium is a fiber, it also regulates the bowels, relieving both constipation and diarrhea. It is imperative that as you kill fungus within the bowels, it is eliminated from the body.

People with gut problems, i.e., constipation, diarrhea, gas, bloating, reflux, etc., almost certainly have an "inflamed" or leaky gut. Psyllium hulls can greatly assist in sealing up the "leaky gut." Once the bowels are moving properly and the intestines are sealed, one can begin to absorb and assimilate nutrients from food. The use of organic foods is then recommended, since these are known to contain more nutrients.

Are psyllium hulls for everyone?

If you suffer from hypertension (high blood pressure), you may take psyllium, but do not take a brand of psyllium hulls that contains licorice, which can elevate blood pressure if taken regularly. Also, if you have any form of intestinal obstruction or have had surgery for intestinal obstruction, please get advice from a health professional prior to taking psyllium hulls.

What are fungi?

How do they differ from bacteria?

Fungi are more highly developed than bacteria or viruses. They range from molds, mushrooms, and tiny round yeast spores to finger or string-like mycelial forms. The number of species of fungi is estimated to be in excess of one million. The number of fungal species implicated in human disease is around four hundred. Some fungi are *dimorphic*, or able to change forms. These can convert from natural, environmental mold forms to invasive round-cell tissue forms. A "*mycoses*" (pronounced 'my-ko-sees') describes a fungal infection of either the skin, deeper tissues, or organs within the human body. No tissue is immune to fungal proliferation.

Fungi (like humans) are heterotrophic, deriving nourishment from organic matter formed by other organisms. For fungi, this can be an animal that has died in the forest, leaves fallen from trees, or you and me! They thrive on warm, moist hosts. Fungi literally live everywhere: the soil, the air, in certain foods, even water. Many fungi are actually residents of the human body in healthy individuals (i.e., in the intestinal tract) and do not cause symptoms or diseases unless the person in which they are living becomes "immunocompromised." The opportunistic fungal organisms can then promote disease by either directly invading the tissues or by producing toxic by-products called *mycotoxins*. Mycotoxins can cause disease even in individuals who were initially healthy.

Bacteria, like fungi, are sometimes also normal residents of the human body. However, their physiology is quite different from fungi. This is why different drugs are used to kill bacteria than those used to kill fungi, though some drugs, sulfa drugs, for example, have both antibacterial and antifungal capabilities. There are harmless "good" bacteria and there are harmful "bad" bacteria. *Lactobacillus acidophilus* is one of several good bacteria that inhabit the small and large intestines and produce chemicals that inhibit the growth of bad bacteria and keep yeast and fungi counts under control. For example, *Lactobacillus acidophilus* produces chemicals that are toxic to the bacteria commonly known to cause "Montezuma's revenge."

It is when these good bacteria succumb to antibiotics, chemicals in food, or chlorinated water that the normal balance is upset and the terrain of the bowel is changed. Without the protective bacteria, yeast can freely proliferate -- this is when normal becomes abnormal and symptoms arise.

lemonade ~ coffee w/stevia ~ water ~ tea
green apple, grapefruit
yogurt ~ cream cheese
egg
oatmeal

chicken, beef
vegetables
brown rice

PHASE ONE

	Included	Excluded
1. Sugar	None	All
2. Artifical or herbal sweetners	Stevia, Stevia Plus	Aspartame, saccharin
3. Fruit	Green apples, berries, avocados, grapefruit, lemons, limes	All others
4. Meat	Fish, poultry, beef, etc.[1]	Breaded meats
5. Eggs	Yes, yolk cooked intact	None excluded
6. Dairy products[2]	Yogurt (including goat yogurt), cream cheese, unsweetened whipping cream, sour cream made with real cream, butter	All others, including margarine and any butter substitutes
7. Vegetables	See note pg. A-24; also, fresh vegetables juiced, including V-8 Juice	Potatoes, yams, legumes (beans and peas)
8. Beverages	Bottled or filtered water, Non-fruity herb teas, Fresh lemonade with stevia	Coffee and tea (including decaf), Sodas (including diet sodas)
9. Grains	None	Pasta, rice, corn, wheat, quinoa, amaranth, millet, buckwheat, oats, barley
10. Yeast products	None	All - including bread, mushrooms, pastries, and alcoholic beverages

-- continued

Phase One, continued

	Included	Excluded
11. Vinegars	Unpasteurized apple cider vinegar, black olives not aged in vinegar	Pickles, salad dressings[3], green olives
12. Oils	Olive, grape seed, flax seed[4], etc. Use cold pressed when available	Partially-hydrogenated oils and peanut oil
13. Nuts	Raw, including pecans, almonds, walnuts, cashews, pumpkin seeds, sunflower seeds, etc.	Peanuts and all peanut products, pistachios

(1) Meat and fish are better if not corn-fed. This means avoiding farm-raised fish.
(2) Dairy products are better if from range-fed cattle.
Good yogurt products: Brown Cow, Monarch Hills, Redwood Hills.
Whipping cream is liquid, unsweetened heavy cream.
(3) Excluded because they are fermented.
(4) Good product: Barlean's

NOTE: Organically grown vegetables are preferable. Meat, eggs, and yogurt should be from animal sources not injected or fed with antibiotics, hormones, or steroids nor fed silo-stored grains.

PHASE TWO

	Included	Excluded
1. Sugar	None	All excluded
2. Artifical or herbal sweetners	Stevia, Stevia Plus	Aspartame, saccharin
3. Fruit	Green apples, berries, avocados, grapefruit, lemons, limes	All others
4. Meat	Fish, poultry, beef, etc.[1]	Breaded meats
5. Eggs	Yes, yolk cooked intact	None excluded
6. Dairy products[2]	Yogurt (including goat yogurt), cream cheese, unsweetened whipping cream, sour cream made with real cream, butter	All others, including margarine and any butter substitutes
7. Vegetables	See note pg. A-26; also, fresh vegetables juiced, including V-8 Juice; *legumes (beans and peas)*	Potatoes, yams
8. Beverages	Bottled or filtered water, Non-fruity herb teas, Fresh lemonade with stevia	Coffee and tea (including decaf), Sodas (including diet sodas)
9. Grains	*Oats (oatmeal), brown rice, quinoa, amaranth, millet, buckwheat, barley; flour tortillas; toasted Sourdough bread[3]*	Corn and wheat

-- *continued*

Phase Two, continued

	Included	Excluded
10. Yeast products	None	All excluded, including bread (except sour-dough), mushrooms, pastries, and alcoholic beverages
11. Vinegars	Unpasteurized apple cider vinegar, black olives in water	Pickles, salad dressings[4], green olives
12. Oils	Olive, grape seed, flax seed[5], etc. Use cold pressed when available.	Partially-hydrogenated oils and peanut oil
13. Nuts	Raw, including pecans, almonds, walnuts, cashews, pumpkin seeds, sunflower seeds, etc.	Peanuts and all peanut products, pistachios

(1) Meat and fish are better if not corn-fed. This means avoiding farm-raised fish.
(2) Dairy products are better if from range-fed cattle.
  Good yogurt products: Brown Cow, Monarch Hills, Redwood Hills.
  Whipping cream is liquid, unsweetened heavy cream
(3) Wheat allergy is common; experiment carefully.
(4) Excluded because they are fermented.
(5) Good product: Barlean's

Italicized Items show additions and changes from Phase One to Phase Two diet.

NOTE: Organically grown vegetables are preferable. Meat, eggs, and yogurt should be from animal sources not injected or fed with antibiotics, hormones, or steroids nor fed silo-stored grains.

Food Facts

There are always hidden ingredients in prepared foods. The following lists will assist you in spotting those ingredients that should be EXCLUDED from your diet. Investigate and *read all labels*!

DAIRY

cow's milk
casein
caseinate
sodium caseinate

whey
lactalbumin
lactalbumin phosphate
buttermilk or buttermilk
    solids

The food industry also produces "Non-Dairy" or "Dairy Free" products; these should also **not** be included in the diet.

SUGAR

lactose (milk/dairy)
sucrose
glucose
maltodextrose
maltose
dextrose

fructose
corn syrup
corn syrup solids
honey [1]
maple syrup

Artificials sweeters should also be excluded from the diet. These are Nutra-Sweet, aspartame, and saccharin/saccharine.

-- continued

VINEGARS

catsup/ketchup	pickles	green olives
mustard	pickled peppers	horseradish
BBQ sauce	hot sauce	dips
soy sauce	salad dressings	mayonnaise
Worcestershire sauce		

These items have been fermented and should be excluded.

YEAST

Hydrolyzed yeast is an additive in many products such as canned and powdered soups and frozen dinners. *Look for it*!

Note:

(1) Honey could be an occasional exception, since it does have some antifungal properties.

Good Food Choices
VEGETABLES

alfalfa sprouts
artichoke, Chinese
asparagus
bamboo sprouts
banana peppers
Bavarian endive
  (escarole, chicory escarole)
bean sprouts
beets
beet greens
bell pepper (sweet green & red)
Brussels sprouts
cabbages --
  bok choy
  broccoli
  cabbage kraut
  cauliflower
  celery cabbage
  Chinese cabbage
  collard greens
  head (green, red)
  kale
  kohlrabi
  savoy
capers, without vinegar
cardoon
carrots
chayte
celery
celeriac (celery root, knob celery)
cucumber
curly endive (chicory)

dandelion greens
dulse
eggplant
fennel (finoccio)
garden cress
garlic
kelp (seaweed)
Lamb's Quarters
leeks
lettuces --
  butterhead
  bib
  Boston
  celtuce (stem)
    iceberg (crisp head)
  loose-leaf
    Lamb's
    matchless
    Oakleaf (green bronze)
    Prizehead
    salad bowl
red leaf chicory --
  arugula
  Romaine (cos)
roguette
rutabaga
onion
okra
parsnip
pumpkin
radish

- *continued*

Vegetables, continued

sea kale
shallot
spinach
squashes --
  acorn
  alligator
  banana
  Boston marrow
  bush
  buttercup
  butternut
  Caserta
  cheese
  cocozelle
  Connecticut field
  cushaw
  Delicious
  Golden Nugget
  hubbard varieties
  mammoth
  Mirliton
  pumpkin
  quaker pie
  Queensland
  straightneck
  Table Queen
  Turbin Virginian
  whitebush scallop
  zucchini
Swiss chard

tomatillo
tomatoes, all kinds
turnip greens
upland cress
water cress
Whitloff chicory (Belgian or
      French endive)
yucca

**Miscellaneous**

agar-agar
aloe vera
carrageen (Irish moss)
pepino (melon pear)
rhubarb

MEATS

beef
  bologna
  liver
  sausage
  milk product: plain yogurt
buffalo
goat (kid) -- milk, cheese
lamb
pork --
  ham
  sausage, etc.
poultry --
  chicken & chicken eggs
  dove
  duck & duck eggs
  goose & goose eggs
  guinea hen
  pea fowl
  pheasant
  prairie chicken
  quail
  turkey & turkey eggs
sea food --
  crustaceans:
    cray fish
    Dungeness crab
    lobster
    shrimp (prawn)
    snow crab
  mollusks:
    clam
    oyster

sea food --
  mollusks, continued:
    scallop
    snail
    squid
  fresh water fish:
    beluga
    carp
    catfish
    caviar (roe)
    crapapie (crappie)
    pickerel
    salmon
    smelt
    sturgeon
    trout, all species
    white & yellow perch
    whitefish
    yellow bass
  salt water fish:
    albacore tuna
    anchovy
    bluefish
    cod (scrod)
    flounder
    haddock
    halibut
    Mahi-Mahi
    ocean catfish
    ocean perch
    pilchard (sardine)

- *continued*

Meats, continued

sea food --
    salt water fish, continued:
        red snapper
        sea bass
        sea herring
        swordfish
        tuna
veal
venison (deer)

Miscellaneous **Not recommended for frequent consumption due to processing and fermentation. Processing can include starch fillers and sugars.**

    bologna
    frankfurters
    sausage
    salami

HERBS & SPICES

allspice
althea root (tea)
angelica
anise
apple mint
balm
basil
bergamot
boneset (tea)
borage
burdock root (tea)
burnet (cucumber flavor)
caraway
cardamom
cassia
celery seed
chamomile (tea)
chervil
chicory (in tea)
chive
cilantro/coriander
clove
comfrey (tea)
cumin
dittany
dry mustard
East Indian arrowroot
fenugreek
ginger
ginseng (tea)
goldenrod (tea)

hibiscus, roselle (tea)
horehound
horseradish
lavender
lemon balm (Melissa)
licorice
lovage
mace
marjoram
menthol
mint
nutmeg
oregano
paprika/paprica
parsley
peppercorns (black, white)
peppermint
pimento
rosemary
saffron
sage
savory
sorrel (dock)
spearmint
tarragon
thyme
turmeric

Miscellaneous
sea salt

IPD Phases One and Two

MENUS

Doug Kaufmann's Favorite Meal!

<u>Dice</u>: tomatoes, onions, cucumbers, avocado, and black olives.

<u>Add</u>: hard-boiled eggs and either smoked salmon or cubes of beef purchased from a health food market.

<u>Toss</u>. <u>Add</u> two tablespoons of olive or grape seed oil and the juice from a freshly-squeezed lemon as the dressing.

Enjoy !

<u>The following pages include recipes for</u>:

Salad & Appetizer
Condiments & Dips
Side Dishes
Main Dishes

Salad & Appetizer

Spinach Salad

1 bunch spinach, torn or
   sliced to desired size
1 cucumber, sliced
2 eggs, hard boiled, sliced

1/2 to 1 c. cauliflowerettes (opt.)
1 - 2 stalks celery, chopped (opt.)
6 radishes, sliced (opt.)

Toss together all ingredients. Flavor as desired with herbs and spices. Serve with lemon and oil dressing. Fresh sprouts or 1/4 cup roasted sunflower seeds may be added to give extra crunch.

Nine Vegetable Cocktail

1 pint fresh tomatoes
1 cucumber, sliced
1 radish, quartered
1/4 onion, sliced

1 green pepper, sliced
1 lettuce leaf
a few sprigs parsley
1 pt. ice cubes, to desired consistency

Optional: 1 slender carrot, 1 stalk celery

In an electric blender, blend together all ingredients adding ice cubes a few at a time. If juice tends to freeze, allow to run a little longer before adding remaining ice. If desired, add salt and pepper or other herbs and spices. Add more ice for colder or thinner juice.

Makes 1-1/2 quarts.

Condiments & Dips

Almost Tartar Sauce

1/2 c. green onions, tops and all,
    coarsely chopped
1/4 c. parsely, no heavy stems,
    coarsely chopped
1/4 c. cucumber, finely chopped
1 tsp. capers

1 tsp. sea salt
1/4 tsp. pepper
1/4 to 1/2 tsp. Mrs. Dash
juice of 1/2 to 1 freshly squeezed
    lemon
1 pt. plain yogurt

Combine all ingredients except yogurt in a bowl and toss to blend. Put mixture through a meat grinder using the coarse blade, or use a blender on 'chop.' Stir mixture into yogurt. Chill.

Serve with fish or with slices, chunks, or cubes of any vegetable.

Basic Vege-Yogurt Dip

1/2 c. plain yogurt
juice of 1/2 lemon

spices and herbs as desired
sea salt to taste

Spices and herbs might include garlic, chives, marjoram, or thyme. Mix together all ingredients. Chill and serve.

Herb Dressing

1 tsp. dry mustard
1 tsp. dill weed
1/4 tsp. tarragon
pinch thyme
pinch oregano

1 Tbsp. fresh parsley, chopped
1/2 tsp. sea salt
1/4 tsp. freshly ground black pepper
1/2 c. virgin olive oil

Stir together all ingredients except olive oil until dry mustard is dissolved. Allow to sit for ten minutes. Blend in olive oil, beginning with 1/3 cup and adding additional oil to taste.

Use to dress green salads or serve with slices, chunks, or cubes of any vegetable.

Condiments & Dips, continued

Mexican Relish

1 lb. tomatillos, peeled
2 pinches cumin
1/2 onion, minced

1 clove garlic
2 serrano chilis

Blend together all ingredients. Melt 1/2 Tbsp. butter in a skillet. Sautee mixture until onions and tomatillos are clear. Serve with chicken, fish, or other vegetables.

Store in the refrigerator.

Salad Dressing and Vegetable Marinade

1/2 c. olive oil
juice of 2 lemons

1 tsp. oregano
1 tsp. garlic powder

Mix together all ingredients in a pint jar. Finish filling the jar with water. Shake well to mix, then pour over vegetables which are whole or have been sliced, chunked, or chopped. Marinate in refrigerator two hours or longer. Other herbs and spices may be added to flavor as desired.

Some vegetables from which to choose are squash, radishes, cucumbers, broccoli, carrots, bell pepper, cauliflower, or onions.

If using on spinach or lettuce, add just prior to serving.

Side Dishes

Curried Cauliflower

1 - 2 c. cauliflowerettes	1/2 tsp. butter
1 onion, thinly sliced	1 tsp. curry powder, or to taste
1/2 c. fat-skimmed chicken stock	1/2 tsp. cumin (opt.)

Combine ingredients in a small pan, cover. Simmer until most of the liquid has evaporated.

Note: Other vegetables may be "curried" in this manner.

Deviled Eggs

6 hard boiled eggs, halved lengthwise	paprika to taste
	2 tsp. dry mustard
salt and pepper to taste	2 Tbsp. plain yogurt

Separate yolks from egg whites. Mash yolks together in a small bowl. Add remaining ingredients, mixing well. Refill egg whites with yolk mixture. Arrange on a platter and sprinkle with additional paprika.

Main Dishes

Beef Patties

1 lb. ground beef
1/2 tsp. sea salt
1/8 tsp. garlic powder
1/4 tsp. black pepper

1 c. onion, finely chopped
- or -
2 tsp. dried onion

Mix together all ingredients. Shape into six patties. Broil or grill to desired doneness.

Optional: Ground chicken, turkey, or lamb may be used in place of beef. If lamb is used, add a pinch of oregano.

Chicken Stroganoff

2 Tbsp. olive oil
1 lb. chicken, chopped or ground
1 med. onion, chopped
1 clove garlic, minced (opt.)
1 c. chicken broth

1 tsp. sea salt
1/4 tsp. pepper
1/2 tsp. thyme
fresh parsley, chopped

Heat oil in a wide frying pan over medium to high heat. Lightly brown the chicken. Just as chicken begins to brown, add onion and garlic, stirring until onion becomes limp and translucent. Add broth, salt, pepper, and thyme. Simmer, stirring frequently until thickened. Serve with brown rice. Garnish with fresh parsley.

Fish Fillet Almondine

1/4 c. olive oil or butter
3 Tbsp. slivered almonds
2 lbs. fish fillets (snapper, cod, sole)

1 Tbsp. lemon juice
1/2 tsp. garlic salt
1/4 tsp. pepper

Heat 2 Tbsp. oil in large skillet. Add almonds and sautee 2 to 3 minutes, stirring constantly, until golden brown. Remove almonds and set aside. In remaining oil, cook fish 3 to 4 minutes on each side until fish flakes when pierced with fork. Remove to warm platter. Add lemon juice, salt, pepper , and almonds to pan drippings; spoon over fish.

Main Dishes, continued

Lemon-Fried Chicken

1 fryer chicken, skin removed
1/4 c. fresh lemon juice
1/4 tsp. garlic salt
3/4 tsp. sea salt
1/4 tsp. thyme

1/4 tsp. marjoram
1/8 tsp. pepper
1/2 tsp. grated lemon rind
2 Tbsp. butter

Cut chicken into serving pieces and place in a large, shallow pan. Mix together the remaining ingredients, except the butter. Pour mixture over the chicken pieces and marinate in the refrigerator for at least three hours, turning occasionally. Drain chicken on absorbent paper.

Preheat skillet, add butter. Add chicken and cook for 15 minutes with lid partially on. Turn chicken and continue cooking for 10 minutes with lid partially on. Place cover on tightly and cook for 15 minutes more. Total cooking time is 30 minutes.

Note: If you use a skillet capable of "greaseless frying," do not add butter.

Mexican Fish

1 - 2 lbs. fish, whole or fillets
1 clove garlic, freshly chopped
1 lime, freshly juiced
pepper to taste, white or black
1 small onion, chopped

1 lb. peeled tomatillos (Mexican
    green tomatoes)
2 pinches cumin
1 clove garlic
1/2 onion, minced
2 serrano chilis (opt.)

Pierce fish on each side with fork. Rub garlic into fish, pour fresh lime juice on inside and outside of fish, then sprinkle with pepper. Marinate two hours. Place, with chopped onion, in cold skillet that maintains an even temperature. Leave on medium heat eight minutes, turn fish over, and cook until done, approximately ten minutes more.

Blend together remaining ingredients. Heat in separate skillet until onion and tomatillos are clear. Pour onto warm platter and top with cooked fish.

Note: this recipe contains no salt. The garlic and lime make salt unnecessary.

Main Dishes, continued

Old Fashioned Pot Roast

3 lb. lean brisket of beef
1 clove garlic, minced
1/2 tsp. black pepper, coarsely
  ground

1 large onion, chopped
1 small bay leaf
1/2 tsp. sea salt
optional vegetables, cut in pieces

Preheat oven to 450 degrees. Rub meat with garlic and pepper; place in a greased Dutch oven or heavy saucepan. Brown for 10 minutes on each side. Slowly and carefully add 1 cup water and remaining ingredients. May also add cleaned, cut vegetables such as carrots, celery, bell peppers, or rutabaga for a simple, one dish meal.

Reduce oven temperature to 300 degrees. Cover and bake 3 hours or until tender.

Makes approximately 10 servings.

Turkey Salad

1 c. turkey, cooked and diced
2 c. rice, chilled
1 c. celery, diced
1 med. green pepper, shredded
1 Tbsp. pimento, chopped

2 Tbsp. parsley, chopped
1/2 c. olive oil
1/3 c. lemon juice
1/2 tsp. curry

Mix together turkey, rice, and vegetables; chill. Combine oil, lemon juice, and curry; let stand for 1 hour. Pour dressing over salad just before serving.

Main Dishes, continued

Tuna Salad

1/2 c. plain yogurt
1 Tbsp. lemon juice
1/4 tsp. sea salt or Mrs. Dash
jalapeno pepper, chopped (opt.)

1 12-oz. can tuna, crumbled
1 small onion, sliced
1 stalk celery, coarsely chopped

Lightly blend all ingredients. Chill and serve with slices, chunks, or cubes of any vegetable.

Makes approximately 1-1/2 cups.

NOTES

APPENDIX B

Product Information

Bio-Active Nutrients
1-800-879-6504

Chromium Picolinate, Caprylic Acid and Glutamine powder.

Carol Bond Health Foods
1-800-833-8282

Geri-Hi, MEGi-Hi, Thistlex, Injuv and Prostate Management.

First Fishery Development Services, Inc.
Seagate – 1-888-505-GATE

Self-manufactured health products, including olive leaf, grape seed extract, shark cartilage, organic carrot powder, garlic powder, and beta glucans.

Natren, Inc.
1-800-992-3323

Healthy Trinity and numerous other probiotic products.

Primal Nutrition
1-888-396-6696

Master Formula vitamins.

Texas TKO
1-866-660-6909

Organic solution to toxic cleaners.

SF722 and all other products mentioned within this work should, at the
time of publication, be available at health food or drug stores.

Index

A

discharge 157
disease, incurable 47
disease, vascular 3
diseases, fungal. *See fungal diseases*
disorders, estrogenic 33
disorders, respiratory 51
dissemination 165
dissemination, bacterial 36
dissemination, fungal 36
drugs, sulfa A-20
duodenitis/proximal jejunitis syndrome (DPJ) 84
dypsnea 55
dysbiosis 138

E

eating disorders 93
eczema 101, 105, 134
Edison, Thomas 124
eggs 108, 119, A-14, A-15
endometriosis 68, 147, 148
energy, loss 86
environment 159
eosinophilia-myalgia syndrome (EMS) 88
Epstein-Barr virus 169
estrogen 155
ethanol 83
exercise A-18
exercise program 77
extra-intestinal symptoms 35
eyes 35

F

farmers lung 12
fatigue 18, 71, 157
fermentation 13
fertility drugs 146
fever 35, 167, A-16
fiber A-7, A-18
fibroids 155
fibromyalgia 6, 167, 174
fistulas, anal 45
Flagyl 45
flora 12, 36

G

gas 149, A-19
gastroenterologist 29
gastrointestinal problems 18
genetics 86
Glaspy, John, M.D. 146
glucose A-5
Gottschalk, Howard, M.D. 129
Gottschall, Elaine 36
gout 17
grains 33, 34, 84, 85, 118, 139, 146, 154
granuloma 119
granulomatous lesions 37
grape seed extract 112, A-9
grapefruit extract, nasal spray 139
gut diseases 27, 36
gut lumen 99
gut problems 27, A-19
gut yeast 39
gynecologist 150

H

hair loss 71
hangover 83
hardening of the arteries. *See atherosclerosis*
Hattersley, Joseph 119
hawthorne berries 112
hay 118
hay fever. *See allergic rhinitis*
HDL 120
headache 71, 164, 167
headaches 18
Healthweek magazine 11
hearing loss 21
heart attack 3, 111, 115, 119, 125
heart disease 111, 165
heartburn 84
Heaton, K. W. 36
Hellinghausen, Mary Ann 11
herbs 140
herniated disc 174
herpes zoster 169
Herxheimer's reaction 71, A-15
heteotrophic A-20
high blood pressure. *See hypertension*

T

U

V